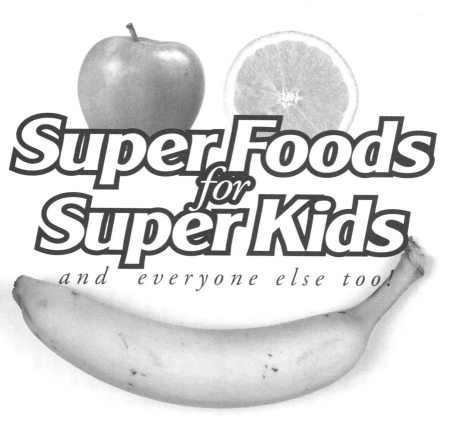

# Super Foods
*for*
# Super Kids
*and everyone else too!*

*35* Nutritious, Delicious Meals *to* Introduce
Your Child *to a* Lifetime *of* Vibrant Health

# VALERIE SAXION, N.D.

## *Super Food for Super Kids*

Copyright © 2003 Valerie Saxion

All Scripture quotations, unless otherwise indicated, are taken from the *Holy Bible, New International Version®*. NIV®. Copyright © 1973, 1978, 1984 by International Bible Society. Used by permission of Zondervan Publishing House. All rights reserved.

ISBN 1-932458-03-4

Published by Bronze Bow Publishing Inc., 2600 E. 26th Street, Minneapolis, MN 55406

You can reach us on the internet at www.bronzebowpublishing.com

Literary development and cover/interior design by
Koechel Peterson & Associates, Inc., Minneapolis, Minnesota.

Manufactured in the United States of America

*To the family that gave me the experience to write this book.
To the best husband and children in the world—my gifts from God!
Jim, your flair for spice is extra nice. Zach the fanatic is the health
nut who at seven years old makes me know raising children the
right way pays off.*

*You all have gone through a lot of trial and error. You've sometimes
even felt as though you live in the dark ages because I won't have a
microwave in the house. Not to mention the various ridicule when
your friends can't identify your lunch!*

*Your love and encouragement drive me to press on to be a Proverbs 31
woman. Without you I would never have made thousands of healthy
school lunches! My love and dedication to Jim, Cortney, Whitney, Lexie,
Hamilton, Morgan, Jesse, Zachary, and Seth.*

*I love you all,*

*Mom*

**DR. VALERIE SAXION** is one of America's most articulate champions of nutrition and spiritual healing. A twenty-year veteran of health science with a primary focus in naturopathy, Valerie has a delightful communication style and charming demeanor that will open your heart, clear your mind, and uplift you to discover abundant natural health God's way. Her pearls of wisdom and life-saving advice are critical for success and survival in today's toxic world.

As the co-founder of Valerie Saxion's Silver Creek Labs, a premier manufacturer and distributor of nutritional supplements and health products that cover a wide range of healing modalities, Dr. Saxion has seen firsthand the power of God's remedies as the sick are healed and the lame walk. "It's what I love most about what God has called me to do," she says.

Valerie Saxion is the host of TBN's *On Call*, which airs twice weekly across America. The program is dedicated to bringing the most up-to-date health and nutritional information to the viewing audience. Dr. Saxion is one of TBN's favorite speakers and can be seen quarterly on the flagship show, *Praise the Lord*. The audience is nationwide as well as international, with a potential 33 million broadcast households.

She is also seen on the Daystar Television Network and Cornerstone Television Network. Dr. Saxion has been interviewed on numerous radio talk shows as well as television appearances nationwide and in Canada. Hosts love to open the line for callers to phone in their health concerns while Dr. Saxion gives on-the-air advice and instruction.

She has also lectured at scores of health events nationwide

and in Canada. She has advised international government leaders, professional athletes, television personalities, and the lady next door. "All with the same great results," she says, "if they will only follow the recommendations."

After attending one of Dr. Saxion's lectures, you may have cried, you may have laughed, you may get insight, but one thing is sure: You will leave empowered with the tools to live and love in a healthy body!

Dr. Saxion is also the author of *How to Feel Great All the Time* and *Every Body Has Parasites* as well as four very practical, life-changing booklets, including *How to Stop Candida and Other Yeast Conditions in Their Tracks, The Easy Way to Regain and Maintain Your Perfect Weight, Conquering the Fatigue, Depression, and Weight Gain Caused by Low Thyroid,* and *How to Detoxify and Renew Your Body From Within.* She is currently a monthly columnist for BeautyWalk.com, hosted by Peter Lamas, famous makeup artist and hair designer for the rich and famous.

Married to Jim Saxion for twenty-plus years, they are the parents of eight healthy children, ages toddler to mid twenties.

To schedule Dr. Saxion for a lecture or interview, please contact Joy at 1-800-493-1146, or fax 817-236-5411, or email at valeriesaxon@cs.com.

As FAR AS I AM CONCERNED, this is the most important book I have written. What we put in the mouths of our children today will shape a generation tomorrow. Are we raising healthy, vibrant youth, or are we raising sickly, immune-suppressed children who pay regular visits to doctors and are dependent on medications to keep them from getting out of hand? I'm afraid it's too often the latter.

Almost twenty years ago I heard Dr. Dobson from *Focus On the Family* say that children who are addicted to sweets today will be the adults who are addicted to drugs and alcohol tomorrow. I often wondered why that was. Today, I agree that addictive personalities may play a role, but I lean more toward the belief that the culprit is Candida Albicans, a parasitic yeastlike fungus that exists naturally in the body and usually causes no bad effects. But if a child's diet is heavy in sugary snacks, sodas, and processed foods, and if the child is given too many antibiotics that kill off the good bacteria as well as the bad bacteria in the body, a yeast overgrowth can happen. Then as the child gets older, the overgrown yeast and parasites drive him or her on to not only sugar addictions but to the yeast in alcohol and much, much more.

Mom and Dad, you can do something about it, and you don't have to have a degree in nutrition to figure it out. You're starting in the right place! *Super Foods for Super Kids.*

If you start where you are and make gradual changes, I have great confidence that you will soon be making the right choices for your family on a daily basis. You are responsible for your family's health—not your doctor or your insurance company. And it starts with the hole below your nose!

You and your children can start saying, "I feel great all the time."

I love and truly appreciate you. God wants you healthy, and so do I.

Many Blessings,

Valerie Saxion, N.D.

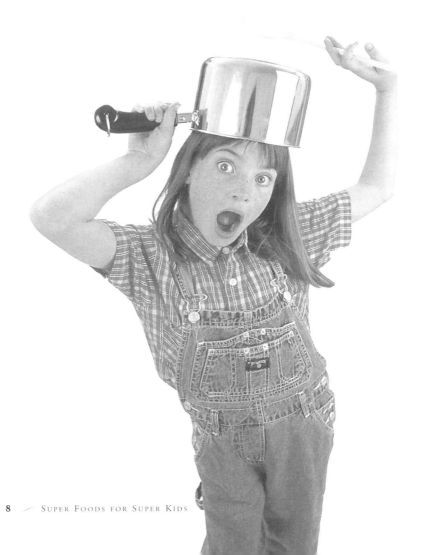

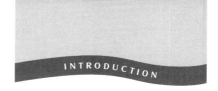
*"My people are destroyed from lack of knowledge."* HOSEA 4:6

**I** RECENTLY RECEIVED THIS MESSAGE from a desperate mother, but I hear echoes of its message wherever I go: "Dear Dr. Saxion, my little boy is already obese. His pediatrician is very concerned but hasn't offered any suggestions other than a modified diet. My son has horrible eating habits, and I have not been able to get him to eat nutritious foods. Sometimes I let him go to bed hungry because he only wants Happy Meals and chips. What do you have that will help him? I will work into my budget *anything* that will help him."

We all want the best of health and well-being for ourselves, and we especially want it for our children. The media has pounded us with the news that the nutritional quality of the diet we provide our kids is the key to supporting their healthy development and directly influences their biochemistry as well as their immune system. Health and nutrition go hand in hand. Whether it involves bacteria, viruses, or fungi, there are many harmful microorganisms that constantly work to suppress the immune system. This can leave our kids more vulnerable to getting sick and make them susceptible to many diseases. The prevalence of the flu and colds and mononucleosis and bronchitis and yeast infections represents but a fraction of the problem faced today by our kids. It is said that by eating just 3 tablespoons of sugar you compromise your immune system up to 6 hours.

But the same media that stresses the importance of nutritious foods also constantly bombards us and our children with advertisements that are designed to mislead. The television ad for our kids' favorite cereal stresses that it is fortified with vitamins and iron and will maintain strong bones . . . but fails to mention that it is loaded down with nearly 40 percent sugar! Walk down the grocery aisle and check out the words on the front of the containers, then go to the back and discover the full story. You'll find that "low fat" is a relative term that should never be trusted, and that "light" probably means that the sugar has been replaced by an artificial sweetener that has its safety questioned by many experts. Is it surprising that manufacturers leave you to figure out that their "power" drink is laced with well over 60 percent sugar?

It doesn't require a doctor to figure out where the confusion comes from, and why there has been a breakdown in the health of today's children. Statistics from the United States Department of Agriculture show that as many as one out of every two Americans is not getting the minimum RDAs (Recommended Dietary Allowances) from their current diet. Keep in mind that these guidelines were established as a minimal level, not for maximizing your health! Meanwhile, other statistics show that fat consumption has increased by 30 percent and sugar consumption by 50 percent in the past several decades. It's a formula ripe for disease and obesity. Over 16 percent of children nationwide are overweight and that percentage is expected to rise.

The Centers for Disease Control and Prevention recently announced that one in three U.S. children born in 2000 will become diabetic unless many more people start eating less and exercising more. The Center also recently stated that obesity is almost the number one health threat in America (tobacco remains the largest cause of death). Dr. Robert Eckol of the American Heart Association reports that a new study shows that "If you're overweight, you basically live three years less . . . and if you're obese, you live approximately six to seven years less." Your family does not need to be a part of these grim statistics.

## Why Nutrition Is So Important

You are mistaken if you think your children are in good health today because they are free from disease. If you are trying to get by with an unbalanced diet, a child's body may be able to cope with a lack of a specific nutritional substance for a while, but you can only cheat for so long and not have them pay a price. Eventually their system will not be able to rid itself of disease, and a health problem will surface. We cannot escape the fact that if we fail to supply their bodies with what they require to maintain the health of their cells, they will reap disease.

Besides the harm being done to children's bodies through poor diet habits and lack of exercise, there are other factors constantly warring against them—most of which we cannot control. The effects of breathing in smog and cigarette smoke, exposure to increasing levels of UV rays, and contact with chemical products as well as their fumes have been shown to cause damage to body cells. We are surrounded by pesticides, asbestos, formaldehyde (in particle board, plywood, paints, and plastics), vinyl chloride, radioactivity, and X-rays—all of which are dangerous.

Add to that the preservatives and chemical additives to food, agricultural pesticides and hormone-enhancing drugs, chemical sprays, food processing, cured and processed meats, and the tremendous amounts of sugar added to our food. Government statistics state that the average American consumes a whopping 120 pounds of sugar each year, which is about 1/3 pound per day. Then there is the health toll from the stresses of daily life—emotional traumas, physical injuries, allergies, antibiotics (that kill both bad and good bacteria in the body), and the fluctuations between hot and cold surroundings. All these negatively affect us and our kids over time, and one might think it a wonder that anyone is healthy.

## Here's Some Really Good News

There is good news, though, despite the bleak picture I've painted. Even if your family's diet has been unbalanced since the day your children were born, God is a God of restoration. He has made the human body in such a wonderful way that it is ceaselessly trying to make and keep itself well. There is hope for every situation . . . even yours. At any moment, 50 percent of the human body's cells are alive, 25 percent are dying off, and 25 percent are dead—this is a phenomenal process of regeneration. The body is making billions of new cells right now. It is so efficient that if a person is eating right, his or her liver will regenerate itself every 7 days. It is actually possible to clean the body quickly and build health back into all the organs.

As long as those new body cells are being manufactured, you can make a difference in your family's health. These cells reach into the bloodstream to obtain more than 50 chemicals: amino acids (the building blocks of protein), fatty acids, minerals, trace elements, vitamins, and enzymes. These chemicals come from the food and water you provide, and the air that is breathed—all of which you can do something about. If you are careful to supply your children with all that they absolutely require for health, whether by nutrients or exercise, radiant health will reign over every aspect of their bodies. They will feel great physically and emotionally! They will have unlimited energy to do all the things they want and to become the persons they want to be.

My hope is that *Super Foods for Super Kids* will help you come to grips with what you are providing or depriving your kids as regards to nutrition. This book will provide you with 35 simple, nutritious meals and over a dozen smoothies your kids will love and that will give their bodies the opportunity to feel great and be truly healthy all of the time. Perhaps you need to start with something as simple as eliminating the junk food from your home and drinking more water in your family. It need not be complicated or expensive, and it doesn't necessitate becoming a vegetarian. It is totally doable, and you can start right where you are today. It begins with simple choices that you have the power to make.

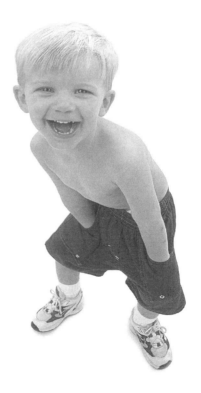

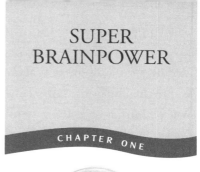

# SUPER BRAINPOWER

CHAPTER ONE

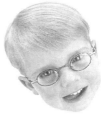

**W**HILE YOUNG BODIES REQUIRE OPTIMAL NUTRITION to propel them vitally through their active days, the brain as the body's most complex organ is the most needy of all. Weighing in at less than three pounds, the brain is the control center of our body's central nervous system. It consists of a compact network of more than ten billion nerve cells, nerve tissue, and nerve-supporting and nourishing tissue (neuroglia). The brain is the center of thought and emotions and regulates bodily activities. It is one of the busiest, most metabolically active organs in the body and is made of approximately 60 percent fat. It is the nutrients in the food we eat that are needed to keep the brain in top working order.

Despite its size, the brain is involved in 15 percent of the body's total blood flow, 25 percent of its oxygen utilization, and at least 70 percent of its glucose (sugar) consumption. Unlike other organs, the brain is not capable of storing its own supply of energy. It depends, rather, on a constant flow of blood for energy. Thus the reason why you get brain fog when you don't eat or don't exercise properly. Good circulation and healthy blood vessels are vital to the feeding of the brain.

Deprived of the proper nutrients in the bloodstream, proteins used by nerve cells in the brain cannot be manufactured, which can lead to the impairment of mental functions such as memory as well as a person's mood. It must have a continual supply of glucose, oxygen, and other essential nutrients. Also, unlike other tissues in the body that can heal after an injury, brain cells are incapable of regenerating themselves. This makes the brain especially vulnerable to illness and injury.

Consider then the importance of this to your child. You hold the keys to the energy that will fuel their brain and which will strongly influence their emotions. Beyond the healthy recipes in this book I will define for you the key nutrients that will provide your child the vital mental building blocks they need to succeed in life. You need to understand the powerful role of proteins, minerals, vitamins, water, carbohydrates, and fats, and how they work together to boost your child's brainpower! Each of these nutrients contributes to the feeding of the brain, and it is up to you to learn the best brain foods and shape your family's diet to the best. It's really not that complicated, so please don't stop with the recipes. Your child's well-being depends on it!

One other crucial point regards you child's sleep. According to a recent report, studies show that children who get an hour more of sleep a night can raise their grades as much as one point. Too many parents allow kids to get away with a lot less sleep than they actually need. And few parents know that girls need at least an hour more sleep than boys. You can provide the best food that money can buy, but nothing takes the place of a good night's rest. That's true for children as well as adults.

## BLACK BEAN ROLL-UPS

1 package tortillas
1 15-ounce can black beans
1 jar favorite salsa
1 avacado
Sea salt

Pepper
Sour cream
1 cup shredded mozzarella cheese
Olives, optional

Scoop out the avacado, mash with fork, add sea salt and pepper to make your own guacamole. Drain black beans, smash with fork or blender. Spread onto tortilla, top with thin layer of homemade guacamole, then add thin layer of salsa and sour cream. Sprinkle with shredded cheese and olives. Carefully roll tortilla and secure with a toothpick. Leave whole or refrigerate 1 hour and slice into bite-size snacks.

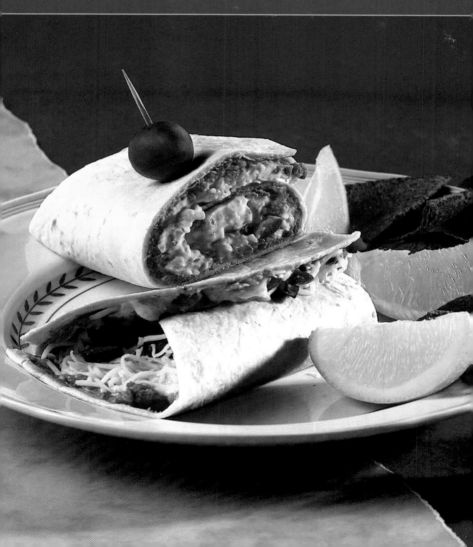

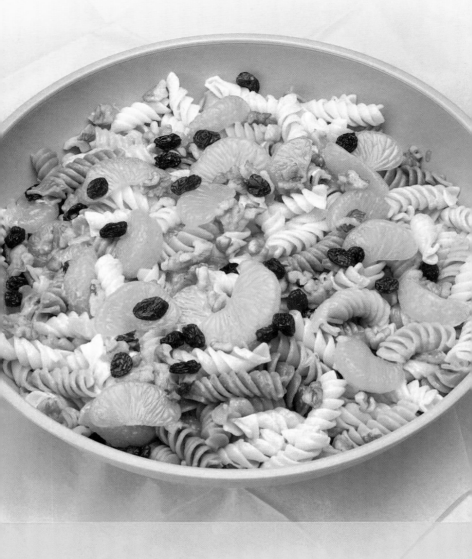

## *FRUITY PASTA SALAD*

1 16-ounce package spiral vegetable pasta, cook as directed with 2 tablespoons extra virgin olive oil and 1/2 teaspoon sea salt. Drain and add the following:

| | |
|---|---|
| 1 8-ounce can mandarin oranges, drained | 1/4 cup chopped walnuts |
| 1/4 cup organic raisins | 1/4 cup natural mayonnaise |

Mix thoroughly.

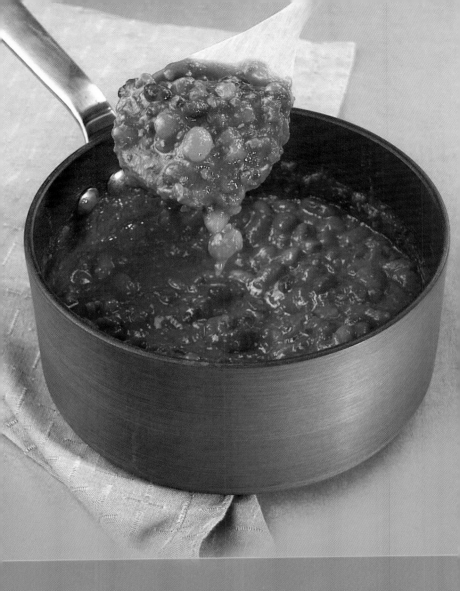

## QUICK VEGETARIAN CHILI

1 can vegetarian chili

Vegetarian chili is easy to find at most health food stores. Open and store in easy to heat bowls for kids to take with them to school.

## HAMILTON'S ZESTY OPEN FACE GUACAMOLE TOAST

Guacamole spread
Vine-ripened tomatoes, sliced
Healthy bread

Toast bread. Spread guacamole on toast. Top with thin slice of tomato. Great for lunch at home or an evening snack.

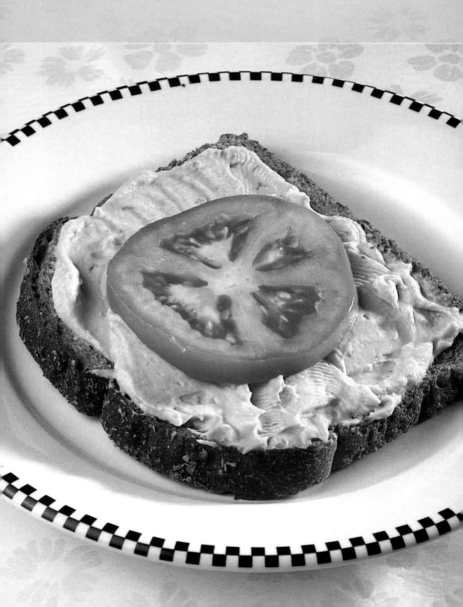

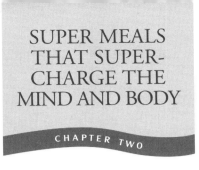

# SUPER MEALS THAT SUPER-CHARGE THE MIND AND BODY

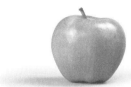

CHAPTER TWO

**THE SCIENTIFIC EVIDENCE** is overwhelming: if you want your family to feel great all the time, you need to make certain they are eating a healthy, energy-packed diet that balances the intake of antioxidants, calcium, complex carbohydrates, essential fatty acids, and proteins. It is important that those foods deliver plenty of fiber, vitamins, and minerals. For most of us it involves moving away from a diet high in processed food, sugar, fat, and meat to a diet that revolves around whole grains, fresh vegetables, and fresh fruits.

The 35 foods that I have selected are super foods that benefit the mind as well as the body. What you eat shapes the health of your cells and organs as well as their ability to function and repair themselves. Nutritional deficiencies cause a breakdown in the building blocks for your body's compounds, hormones, and enzymes. *All* the basic functions of your body, including your brain, are dependent upon an adequate supply of nutrition, and they operate only as efficiently as they are healthy.

My 35 delicious, balanced meals will introduce your kids to a lifetime of vibrant health. And it will provide you with 7 weeks' worth of great meals to replace the empty calories that are routinely served in school cafeterias all over America. You'll spend a minimal amount of time in the kitchen, and the results will be fantastic.

## QUICKIE PROTEIN SNACK OR BREAKFAST

1/2 cup organic cottage cheese (each serving is
   approximately 13–15 grams of protein)
Fresh pineapple cut in bite size or canned without syrup
A drizzle of real maple syrup

This is a tasty snack or quick breakfast that's high in protein. Everybody loves it!

**SUPER FOOD**

**Pineapple** is very juicy and mildly acidic, more like a citrus fruit. They contain a digestive enzyme, bromelain, that allows for their easy digestion. Because of this, pineapples are one of the few fruits that can be eaten following a meal. Bromelain may also have an anti-inflammatory action in the body. Pineapples contain vitamins A and C as well as potassium, calcium, and the trace minerals manganese and selenium. Manganese levels are in fact quite good; one cup of pineapple will supply our minimum daily needs, about 2.5 mg.

## QUICK 10-MINUTE POWER BREAKFAST

Free-range eggs boiled (10 minutes to boil)
Your favorite flavor kefir
Fresh berries
6–8 ounces apple juice
1 ounce liquid minerals
Mix minerals into juice

In this very simple meal, you have a complete protein and whole food in the egg, good bacteria in the kefir, antioxidants in the berries, and all the minerals your body needs in the juice mix. Kefir is an excellent source of good bacteria, but tastes like a milk shake.

**SUPER FOOD**

**Kefir** is a soured and fermented milk product, which is more of a drink than yogurt. It has similar properties, though most kefir available is flavored and sweetened with fruit. It is often a good nutritious substitute for milk, especially for children. Drinking kefir reduces the symptoms of lactose intolerance. Researchers say that kefir contains microbes that carry the enzyme for breaking down lactose. It contains a wider range of bacteria than yogurt, and it's possible it could be even better for your health.

## HAMILTON'S ZESTY OPEN FACE GUACAMOLE TOAST

Guacamole spread
Vine-ripened tomatoes, sliced
Healthy bread

Toast bread. Spread guacamole on toast. Top with thin slice of tomato.
Great for lunch at home or an evening snack.

**Avocados** are unique among the fruits in that they are a very concentrated food, more like a nut than a fruit. They are high in calories—one average avocado has about 300 calories and about 30 grams of fat, as well as 12 grams of carbohydrate and 4 to 5 grams of protein. They are a good source of fat for people who have a problem assimilating other fatty foods. They are fairly high in most of the B vitamins except B12, being particularly good in folic acid, niacin, and pantothenic acid. They also have some vitamin C, good amounts of vitamin A, and contain a bit of vitamin E. Avocados are very rich in potassium and are also particularly good in many other minerals, including magnesium, iron, and manganese. Avocados are commonly used in salads, dips such as guacamole, in sandwiches, or stuffed with seafood.

## ONCE IN A BLUE MOON DOG

1 package Hebrew National Hot Dogs (all-beef kosher
  meat dogs)
Whole grain buns
Condiments

### SERVE WITH:

Crunchy nut granola
Cinnamon applesauce
Lemon ginger tea

**Whole grains** include wheat, rice, oats, corn, barley, rye, millet, buckwheat, spelt, tricale, and quinoa. They satisfy our hunger, provide long-lasting energy, help balance brain chemistry, calm nerves, and encourage deep sleep. They also promote healthy elimination, good memory, clear thinking, and quick reflexes.

## ALMOND BUTTER AND BANANA SANDWICH OR SNACK

Almond Butter
Bananas
Ezekiel bread

Because it has no preservatives, Ezekiel bread is found in the freezer section of your grocery story or health food store. It is sprouted and very healthy. This combination of ingredients makes an awesome sandwich, and it's great brain food as well. Also excellent without bread.

**SUPER FOOD**

**Almond Butter** is made from raw almonds. Almonds are probably the best all-around nut. Their fat content is less than most, about 60 percent, and the protein concentration is nearly 20 percent. They are one of the richest sources of alpha-tocopherol vitamin E. The almond has strong medicinal action including inhibition of cancer. The almond nuts are the fruits of a small tree that grows nearly thirty feet tall and is abundant in many areas of the world, including Asia, the Mediterranean, and North America. Almonds which are of the soft-shell variety possess a sweeter nut than those in hard shells.

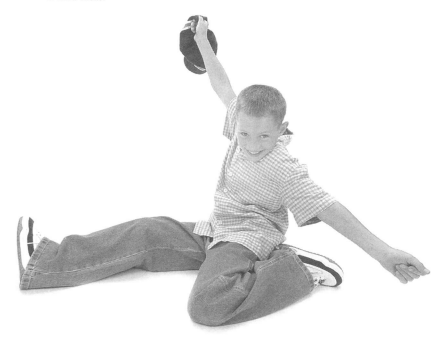

## ROLL-ABLES INSTEAD OF LUNCHABLES

6–8 preservative-free turkey breasts, sliced medium thin
6–8 pieces provolone cheese
Cream cheese
1 cucumber, peeled, sliced, and cubed
Flaxseeds
Toothpicks

Layer, starting on bottom—slices of turkey breast, provolone, and cream cheese. Make a line in the center with cucumber cubes, then sprinkle with flaxseeds. Starting at one side, roll into tight cylinder. Pin with toothpicks.

### SERVE WITH:

All natural Cheetos®
Fresh strawberries
Granola bar
Orange Zinger tea

**SUPER FOOD**

**Flaxseeds** are the richest source there is for the Omega-3 fatty acids. They contain up to 40 percent oil, primarily linoleic and linoleic acids, which are excellent for strengthening the immune system, alleviating rheumatoid arthritis, clearing the heart and arteries, and helping prevent cancer. It has antibacterial, antifungal, and antiviral properties and can be ground and used as a raw condiment or supplement.

## ANN'S HIGH PROTEIN FRUIT SALAD

1 cup organic cottage cheese (26 protein grams)
1 cup plain, vanilla, or organic strawberry yogurt
1 unpeeled apple diced
1 20-ounce can crushed pineapple (unsweetened in own juice), drained
1 banana sliced
1/2 cup organic raisins
1/2 cup chopped pecans

Mix and chill. May add berries in season—blueberries, raspberries, strawberries, and even grapes.

### SERVE WITH:

Barbeque chicken wings or legs
Apple wedges with almond butter
Lemonade

**SUPER FOOD**

**Pecans** are a relative of walnuts and a member of the hickory genus. They are low in sodium and high in most other minerals, including zinc, iron, phosphorus, potassium, selenium, and magnesium. Copper, calcium, and manganese are also present in good amounts. Pecans contain some vitamins A, E, and C, niacin, and other B vitamins. Of all the nuts, pecans are second only to macadamias in fat (over 70 percent) and contain the lowest protein (about 10 percent). Shells should be light brown—if they're red, they've been dyed.

## FRUITY PASTA SALAD

1 16-ounce package spiral vegetable pasta, cook as
directed with 2 tablespoons extra virgin olive oil and 1/2
teaspoon sea salt. Drain and add the following:
1 8-ounce can mandarin oranges, drained
1/4 cup chopped walnuts
1/4 cup organic raisins
1/4 cup natural mayonnaise

Mix thoroughly.

### SERVE WITH:

Barbeque chicken wings or legs
Apple wedges with almond butter
Lemonade

**SUPER FOOD**

**Raisins** are full of iron, potassium, magnesium, phosphorus, and calcium, as well as vitamins A and B-complex. If you take 1 pound of grapes and dehydrate them, you'll have .25 pound of raisins. Raisins are still sun-cured, which enhances their flavor. Unfortunately, raisins contain the highest levels of pesticide residue of any fruit, so buy organic raisins. To keep raisins from becoming dry when baking, plump them in water for 15 minutes before mixing into baked goods.

## CHICKEN SALAD

4–6 chicken breasts, boiled and chopped
4 boiled eggs, chopped
1/4 cup sweet pickle relish
1/2 cup chopped onion
1 Granny Smith apple, chopped with skin
1/2 cup almond slivers
Sea salt to taste
Cracked pepper to taste
Enough mayonnaise to mix

### GREAT SERVED WITH:

Pita bread
Carrot sticks
Dill pickles
Red Zinger tea

**SUPER FOOD**

**Chicken breast** is a wonderfully lean meat that I use all the time. A portion size of 1/2 breast delivers 26 protein grams and only 3 fat grams in contrast to a 3-ounce portion of red meat that brings 23 protein grams and 13 fat grams. The fattiest parts of a chicken are the wings, which have a lot of skin and little meat, and the thighs. Always remove the skin to cut out the fat.

## SALMON SALAD

1 15-ounce can salmon, drained, boned, and skinned
1 bag mixed organic salad greens
1/4 cup sunflower seeds
1 8-ounce can mandarin oranges
1 avocado

Wash and drain greens. Layer greens on bottom of bowl, top with the rest of the ingredients, and drizzle a small amount of dressing over the ingredients.

By the way, I prefer to use my leftover salmon from dinner rather than from a can.

### SERVE WITH:

Ranch dressing
Barbara's Bakery lemon yogurt granola bar
Red delicious apple
Lemon Zinger tea

**SUPER FOOD**

**Sunflower seeds** contain complete proteins with only 20 percent fat, which is mostly unsaturated. As a complete protein, their nutritional value is complete without further preparation. They are a good source of zinc, calcium, phosphorus, and iron, as well as vitamins A, D, E, and several of the B-complex. Whole seeds have a good shelf life, but once hulled they should be refrigerated.

## TURKEY SALAD

2 cups cooked turkey, cut into 1/2" cubes
1/2 cup medium avocados (cut into 1/2" cubes)
1 ripe small tomato, seeded and diced (about 1/2 cup)
2 tablespoons diced red onions
1/4 cup slivered almonds
3 eggs, boiled and diced

Mix ingredients together.

### SERVE WITH:

Whole grain bread or rice cakes or in pita bread
Granny Smith apple
Pretzel sticks
Oatmeal raisin cookie
Bottled water

**SUPER FOOD**

**Red Onions** contain the same potent antioxidant quercitin as other onions, but are a more concentrated source of it. The quercitin, along with the sulphur amino acids also in onions, helps to excrete toxic heavy-metal compounds that build up in the body. Onions also have antibiotic, antiviral, and anti-candida properties. They contain sulfur compounds that lower cholesterol. When eaten regularly, onions are powerful fighters in the war on cancer and heart disease. They are 90 percent water and low in calories.

## EGG SALAD IN A POCKET

3 eggs, boiled and chopped
Nutritious mayonnaise
Sea salt
Relish
Pita bread
Sunflower seeds
Alfalfa sprouts

Combine eggs, mayonnaise, salt, and relish. Fill bottom of pita pocket with egg salad, sprinkle with sunflower seeds, and top with alfalfa sprouts.

### SERVE WITH:

Bugs on a Boat (see recipe on page 52)
Granola bar
Snack bag of grapes
Concord grape juice

**SUPER FOOD**

**Alfalfa sprouts** are up to 30 percent protein by dry weight and are an excellent source of chlorophyll, bioflavonoids, and carotenes. It acts as a laxative, improves the flow of urine, and is rich in nutrients. Almost as good as seaweed as a mineral source, alfalfa contains iron, sulfur, silicon, chlorine, cobalt, magnesium, calcium, potassium, and zinc. It is by far the most common sprout to be in salads or sandwiches. They are very tasty but should be eaten fresh so that they do not ferment.

## SWEET COUSCOUS

1 cup small couscous from bulk
2 cups water
1/2 teaspoon sea salt
1/3 cup organic raisins
2 tablespoons extra virgin olive oil
2 tablespoons pine nuts

In pot, add water, salt, nuts, raisins, and 1 tablespoon oil. Bring to a boil. Add couscous and 1 tablespoon oil. Stir, cover, and remove from heat. Let sit 5 minutes.

## SERVE WITH:

Celery sticks with almond butter
Fresh strawberries with vanilla yogurt for dipping
Yogurt pretzels
Bottled water

**SUPER FOOD**

**Couscous** is a delicious variety of cracked wheat, smaller than the bulgur. It is also used commonly in the Middle Eastern diet—mutton and couscous is the traditional fare in those countries. Couscous is also very good with lentils or chickpeas, and this versatile grain can be used in a main dish, in a salad, or even in desserts. It is easily prepared by pouring boiling water over this soft grain or by lightly cooking. Select couscous that looks fresh and has a fresh aroma and taste. Store in the refrigerator.

## MASHED SWEET POTATOES

2 medium sweet potatoes, baked
1 teaspoon cinnamon
1/4 cup organic raisins
2 tablespoons butter
1/4 cup chopped walnuts

Peel the baked sweet potatoes and mash until smooth. Fold in remaining ingredients. Serve warm.

Loaded with minerals and great any time of the year!

### SERVE WITH:

Baby spinach salad

Sliced turkey breast (I bake a turkey breast every couple of weeks and keep the leftovers for lunches)

Cranberry juice

**SUPER FOOD**

**Sweet Potatoes** is a wonderful source of vitamin E and also contain carotenoids, which are excellent antioxidants. A 5" x 2" baked sweet potato contains more than 2.5 times the U.S. Recommended Dietary Allowance and nearly 30 milligrams of vitamin C, or about a third of what you need in a day. That sweet potato also contributes 3.5 grams of fiber to your diet, all for just 117 calories.

## HEALTHY RICE PILAF

1 cup brown rice (cook as directed,
  with 1/2 teaspoon sea salt)
1/4 cup extra virgin olive oil
1/4 cup chopped onion
1 garlic clove, minced
1/4 cup bean sprouts
1/4 cup dried cranberries or organic raisins
1/4 cup drained peas
1/4 cup slivered almonds

Sauté onion, bean sprouts, garlic, and oil. Add cranberries or raisins and almonds. Toss until coated with oil, then add rice. Mix and serve.

### SERVE WITH:

Chicken fingers with honey

Mandarin oranges

Barbara's Bakery granola bar

Orange Zinger tea

**SUPER FOOD**

**Brown Rice** is not as high in protein as wheat and some other grains, but the protein is very good quality and easily usable. Brown rice has its bran layers intact, and therefore all its nutrients are present. The bran protects the germ's fragile fatty acids. It is better in thiamine, biotin, niacin, pyridoxine, and pantothenic and folic acids than it is in riboflavin and vitamin B12. It has no vitamins A or C, but some vitamin E. Rice, if grown in selenium-rich soil, is very rich in selenium, a scarce but important trace mineral. Magnesium, manganese, potassium, zinc, and iron are all found in good amounts. Sodium is low, but phosphorus, copper, and calcium are all available.

## TUNA PÂTÉ

1 15-ounce can albacore tuna, drained
4 ounces cream cheese
1/4 teaspoon dill weed
1/4 cup chopped purple onions
1/2 teaspoon sea salt
1/4 teaspoon paprika
1/4 cup diced celery
1/4 cup finely chopped walnuts
1/4 cup finely chopped apple
Rice cakes or healthy crackers

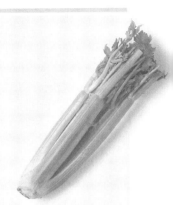

In blender, mix tuna, cream cheese, dill weed, onion, salt, paprika, and celery until smooth. Spread on rice cakes, top with apples and walnuts.

### SERVE WITH:

Mixed raw veggies
Cup of yogurt
Ginger ale

**SUPER FOOD**

**Tuna** is a great source of zinc and the Omega-3 oils (the "good" fat)—a type of polyunsaturated fat associated with a lower risk of heart disease and possibly other diseases. That's why the American Heart Association recommends eating at least two servings of fish per week. A 3-ounce portion of tuna delivers 21 grams of protein with only 0.7 grams of fat. Its firm, light-colored flesh is the only type of tuna that can be labeled as "white meat" on cans. Its flavor is mild compared to other types of tuna. Whether you like canned tuna or not, you might want to try fresh tuna fillets or steaks. Most people say fresh tuna tastes completely different than canned. It can be grilled, broiled, baked, or poached.

## LENTIL SOUP

1 1-pound bag lentils soaked in water for 1 to 2 hours
  or overnight
4 cups chicken stock or broth
4–6 cloves garlic, chopped
1–2 large onions, chopped
1/4 cup grated carrots
1/4 cup extra virgin olive oil
1/2 cup chopped celery
Sea salt to taste
Pepper or cayenne to taste
Enough water for desired consistency

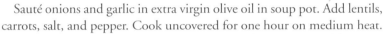

Sauté onions and garlic in extra virgin olive oil in soup pot. Add lentils, carrots, salt, and pepper. Cook uncovered for one hour on medium heat.

For those who like creamy soup, mix 1 cup of milk with 3 tablespoons of corn starch and add to the soup when almost done cooking.

The best way to get the broth for the chicken is to boil 4 to 6 chicken breasts and take out the chicken to use for chicken salad. Reserve the broth for soup. I save all my broth and make the soup really rich and tasty.

After soaking lentils, the cooking is a breeze.

This freezes extremely well, so you can pack individual servings and thaw one at a time.

### GREAT SERVED WITH:

Brown rice salad with dried cranberries and nuts
Celery stuffed with almond butter
Corn muffins (also can be frozen and thawed one at a time)
Lemonade

**SUPER FOOD**

**Lentils** date back to the account in Genesis 25:34 where Esau sold his birthright to Jacob for a tasty bowl of lentil stew. For centuries it has remained a dietary staple across Europe and the Middle East. It ranks just under soy as a top legume protein source, is mild to the taste, and benefits the heart and circulatory systems. They are high in calcium, magnesium, potassium, phosphorus, chlorine, and vitamin A.

## QUICK VEGETARIAN CHILI

1 can vegetarian chili

Vegetarian chili is easy to find at most health food stores. Open and store in easy to heat bowls for kids to take with them to school.

### SERVE WITH:

1 slice of Ezekiel bread

Green salad topped with sunflower seeds, avocado chunks, and almond slivers

Fresh berries in baggie

Bottled water

Because it has no preservatives, Ezekiel bread is found in the freezer section of your grocery story or health food store. It is sprouted and very healthy.

**SUPER FOOD**

**Chili peppers** are a great source of vitamin C and other antioxidant nutrients, including beta-carotene. They have been used widely as natural remedies for coughs, colds, sinusitis, and bronchitis. There is some evidence that chilies help low-density lipoprotein (LDL), or bad cholesterol, and they raise your endorphin level, so you feel better. And they are low in calories while adding fiber and iron to your diet.

## BLACK BEAN ROLL-UPS

1 package tortillas
1 15-ounce can black beans
1 jar favorite salsa
1 avacado
Sea salt
Pepper
Sour cream
1 cup shredded mozzarella cheese
Olives, optional

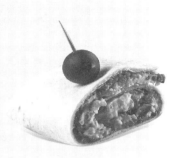

Scoop out the avacado, mash with fork, add sea salt and pepper to make your own guacamole. Drain black beans, smash with fork or blender. Spread onto tortilla, top with thin layer of homemade guacamole, then add thin layer of salsa and sour cream. Sprinkle with shredded cheese and olives. Carefully roll tortilla and secure with a toothpick. Leave whole or refrigerate 1 hour and slice into bite-size snacks.

### SERVE WITH:

Blue corn chips
Orange wedges
Hibiscus tea

**SUPER FOOD**

**Black Beans**, or turtle beans, are members of the kidney bean family and are loaded with proteins. This is excellent protein with none of the hormones, pesticides, antibiotics, and other toxin residues that end up in animal protein. Black beans are sweet and spicy and taste great in soups or refried.

## CHICKEN BURRITOS

1 chicken, boiled or breast-only boiled, deboned,
  and shredded
Extra virgin olive oil
1 medium onion, minced
2 garlic cloves, chopped
1/4 teaspoon sea salt
1 jar salsa
1 cup shredded real cheddar cheese
1 fresh avocado, chopped
1 package whole grain tortillas

In skillet, sauté oil, onion, and garlic until clear. Mix shredded chicken with salt and add mix from skillet. Put medium amount down the center of a tortilla top with salsa and cheese.

I make these as I'm cooking dinner, and I have my kids roll and wrap each one individually, which gets packed in their school lunches the next morning. Keep leftover mix and freeze or add to omelet.

By the way, always keep the chicken broth for soups—refrigerate or freeze.

### SERVE WITH:

Nutritious corn chips
Snack bag of almonds and raisins
Snack bag of orange slices
Ginseng cola

**SUPER FOOD**

**Garlic** has strong antimicrobial power and is more effective against pathogens than most antibiotics today. It is an excellent antioxidant that stimulates the number of immune cells and is antiviral and antiparasitic. Garlic is also a powerful force in reducing cholesterol and triglycerides and promotes the growth of healthy intestinal flora that are a key to health. It contains a compound called S-allylcysteine, which many experts believe contains the vegetable's anticancer agent.

## BARBECUE SANDWICH

1 8-ounce package firm tofu
Extra virgin olive oil
1/2 onion, sliced in rings
Barbecue sauce
Whole grain buns

In pan, sauté onion in extra virgin olive oil. Slice tofu in medium thin slices and add to onions in pan. Cover with barbecue sauce. Heat for 10 minutes. Serve on bun or open face on toast.

### SERVE WITH:

Coleslaw
Baked beans
Oatmeal cookie with raisins and walnuts
Orange Zinger tea

**SUPER FOOD**

**Tofu** is the best known soy food in America and contains a full spectrum of naturally occurring soy isoflavones. It is made of soymilk curdled with nigari or calcium sulfate and takes on the consistency of a firm custard. It is an excellent food for heart health and cancer prevention. Combine it with the whole grain bun and you get an easily digested high-quality protein that is cholesterol-free and low in saturated fats.

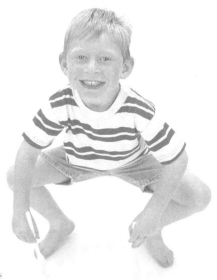

## TURKEY BURGERS

1–2 pounds ground turkey breast
1/2 cup bread crumbs
1/2 cup finely chopped onion
Sea salt
3 eggs
Extra virgin olive oil
Whole grain buns

Combine all ingredients except oil. Shape mix into patties and heat a small amount of oil in skillet. Cook patties through on each side. For those who like a little spice, such as my seven-year-old, Zachary, add a 1/4 cup salsa to mix. Make extra and freeze in individual baggies and take out as needed.

## SERVE BURGER WITH:

Carrot sticks

Dill pickles

Condiments

Applesauce

For a hot meal, serve over brown rice and top with gravy recipe below.

2 cups organic chicken broth
1 cup organic milk or rice milk
3 tablespoons natural corn starch
Sea salt
Pepper
3 tablespoons butter

In skillet, melt butter, add chicken broth, heat through. Mix corn starch with milk and add to broth. As it thickens, add salt and pepper.

*(continued on next page)*

## SERVE RICE AND GRAVY WITH:

Steamed broccoli

Carrot sticks

Spinach salad

**Turkey** is very low in fat, reasonably priced, and may be found in the natural and antibiotic-free state. It contains tryptophan, the essential amino acid that is the building block of serotonin and regulates our metabolism and induces sleep. A 3-ounce portion of turkey delivers 25 grams of protein and only 2 grams of fat.

## VEGGIE BURGER

1 package frozen veggie burgers

Healthy condiments

Swiss or provolone cheese

Whole grain buns

There are many varieties of frozen veggie burgers in your frozen food section or health food store. Cook veggie burgers as directed.

## SERVE WITH:

Dill pickle

Carrot sticks

Apple juice

**Swiss cheese** is fantastic source of calcium, delivering 530 mgs. of calcium for every 2-ounce portion. Our need for calcium is critical during the growth years of infancy and childhood, for building healthy bones and teeth, but is also important lifelong to keep our bones healthy.

## HOMEMADE VEGGIE BURGERS

1 15-ounce can black beans, rinsed, drained, and mashed
1/4 cup shredded carrots
1/2 cup whole kernel corn, drained
1 small onion, diced
1/2 teaspoon sea salt
4 eggs
1/4 cup bread crumbs
Extra virgin olive oil

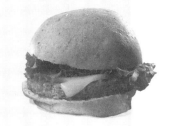

Mix all ingredients except oil. Heat oil in skillet. Shape mixture into small patties and cook through on each side. Drain on paper towel. Serve with guacamole and salsa.

Easy to make extra patties for freezing.

### SERVE WITH:

Carrot, raisin, and pineapple salad
Dill pickles

**SUPER FOOD**

**Carrots** are rich in carotenes and an excellent source of chromium and fiber. Beta-carotene may help prevent cancer of the lungs, cervix, and gastrointestinal tract. Carrots also give your immunity system a boost. A 7"- to 8.5"-long carrot has more than 2,000 mg. of vitamin A—more than twice what you need in a day—and just 30 calories. You also get about 2 grams of fiber and nearly 250 milligrams of potassium. By the way, peeled baby carrots are not really babies. They are adult carrots whittled down.

## *BARBECUE CHICKEN LEGS*

Chicken legs or drumettes
Barbecue sauce

Cover chicken with sauce and bake 20 minutes at 350° F.

### SERVE WITH:

Banana flan pie (see recipe on page 50)
Carrot salad
Yogurt pretzels and yogurt almonds
Bottled water

**SUPER FOOD**

**Bananas** are high in potassium, so they are good for keeping potassium levels up during periods of stress. Bananas are almost completely made up of carbohydrate. They contain many vitamins and minerals, including iron, selenium, and magnesium. Ripe bananas are good for digestive health and can help with constipation and diarrhea. Bananas are used in flavoring for desserts and banana bread, in breakfast cereals, or even in sandwiches. Most commonly, though, they are eaten after peeling the skin as a snack or dessert carried to work or school. As far as treats go, bananas are one of the healthiest, low-calorie snacks.

## *YOGURT/MUSTARD CHICKEN FINGERS*

1–2 pounds chicken breast, boneless, skinless strips
1/2 cup mustard
1 cup plain yogurt
1–2 cups favorite natural crackers, crushed to crumbs
Extra virgin olive oil
Raw honey

Mix yogurt and mustard in bowl. Roll chicken in mixture, then roll in bread crumbs. Pour enough extra virgin olive oil in bottom of pan to coat and lay chicken strips in bottom, 1/2" apart. Bake at 350° F for 20 to 30 minutes.

Serve hot or cold with honey as dip. Kids love it!

### SERVE WITH:

Fruit salad
Applesauce
Bottled water

**SUPER FOOD**

**Yogurt**, or fermented milk, isn't mentioned in the Bible, but according to history we know that it was a mainstay at that time. Yogurt has been attributed to longevity in many civilizations. It is the ideal diet food for folks who want to add flavor and health benefits to their diet. Be sure to get the yogurt with "live" bacterial cultures (*Lactobacillus acidophilus*) and without artificial sweeteners or with added sugars. Yogurt is a natural antibiotic that keeps your digestive system healthy by replacing the good flora in the intestinal track. This is needed for a healthy immune system. You can use yogurt in a variety of ways with salad dressings. It's a healthy snack—my favorite is my *Creation's Bounty* Shake with yogurt in the mornings! Those who are lactose-intolerant typically do fine with a good yogurt.

## CHICKEN CASHEW CROQUETTES

1–2 pounds chicken, boneless, skinless
1/4 cup finely chopped celery
2 tablespoons finely chopped onion
1 cup bread crumbs
3 eggs, beaten
1/4 cup milk
1/2 cup chopped cashews
Extra virgin olive oil
Sea salt and pepper

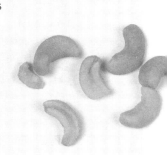

Boil chicken, cut into bite-size pieces. Combine all ingredients with extra virgin olive oil. Heat oil on medium heat. Form patties and sauté on each side for approximately 10 minutes or until browned on each side. Great hot or cold.

### SERVE WITH:

Red grapes
All natural chips
Mango tea

**SUPER FOOD**

**Cashews** are rich in magnesium, potassium, iron, selenium, and zinc. Calcium is lower in cashews than in other nuts, as is manganese; cashews also have a lower fat (47 percent) and higher carbohydrate level than most other nuts. They contain 20 percent protein. Some B vitamins are present, as is vitamin A, though very little vitamin E is found in cashews.

## FAUX CHICKEN PARMESAN

1 box vegetarian chicken patties
Sliced mozzarella cheese
1 jar spaghetti sauce
Optional—whole grain buns
Optional—pasta

Vegetarian chicken patties are found in the freezer section at the grocery store. Heat patties as directed. Heat sauce in small sauce pan. If serving with pasta, prepare pasta as directed. Combine pasta and chicken on a plate and cover with sauce. Top with cheese and heat under broiler until melted.

With bun, prepare chicken and sauce the same and heat under broiler and serve.

### SERVE WITH:

Small garden salad
Apple bread pudding
Bottled water

**SUPER FOOD**

**Mozzarella cheese** is delicious and may be eaten as is with fruit, in sandwiches, or in cooked dishes such as lasagna and pizza. It may also be used as a garnish for salads or other foods. A 1-ounce serving of light mozzarella cheese provides 59 calories, 8 grams of protein, 1 gram of carbohydrate, 2.5 grams of total fat with 2.4 grams of saturated fat, 211 mg. of calcium, 192 mg. of sodium.

## FLAT BREAD PIZZA

1 package Mediterranean flat bread
1 jar favorite healthy salsa
1 cup shredded mozzarella cheese
1/4 cup shredded carrots
Ground-up flax

Lay flat bread out, top with salsa and carrots, sprinkle on flax and top with cheese. Bake for 10 to 12 minutes in preheated oven to 350° F.

### SERVE WITH:

Pineapple sticks
Cucumber rings with ranch dressing
Club soda with cranberry juice (half-and-half mixture)

**SUPER FOOD**

**Mediterranean flat bread** is exactly what it says, flat bread. It does not rise like other bread because it does not have all the yeast. Much like tortillas or pita bread without the pocket, Mediterranean flat bread is wonderful for making wraps. Flat breads are carried in most stores and can be found with all natural organic whole wheat and a variety of other ingredients, including no yeast or salt.

## MORGAN'S VEGGIE STIR FRY

1 15-ounce can whole kernel corn, drained
1/2 medium onion, chopped
2 garlic cloves, minced
1 vine-ripened tomato, chopped and seeded
1 zucchini, peeled and thinly sliced
1 yellow squash, washed and sliced
1 cup fresh spinach
Extra virgin olive oil

In skillet, sauté onions and garlic in oil until clear. Add zucchini and squash and heat until tender. Toss in corn, tomato, and spinach. Continue until spinach is slightly wilted.

### SERVE WITH:

Cold salmon patties or chicken strips

Fresh cherries

Cheese straws

Lemon ginger tea

**SUPER FOOD**

**Tomatoes** are one of the most versatile food ingredients and a staple of the Mediterranean diet. They contain lycopene, a powerful pigment and antioxidant important in the prevention of cancer, as well as significant levels of vitamin E, less of vitamin C, and a small amount of beta-carotene. Tomatoes are a good source of the flavonoid substance quercetin. Canned tomatoes have similar nutritional values, except for lower carotenes and vitamin C. Dried tomatoes and tomato paste are excellent. Look out for the added salt in tomato juice.

## SPINACH QUICHE

1 8-ounce package frozen spinach, cooked and drained
1/4 cup chopped onion
3–4 tablespoons extra virgin olive oil
1/4 teaspoon nutmeg
1 9" deep dish frozen pie crust
3 eggs, beaten
1/2 cup milk
1 1/2 cup shredded Swiss cheese
Sea salt to taste

Sauté onions in extra virgin olive oil and add in beaten eggs and milk. Add cooked spinach, nutmeg, and salt. Mix thoroughly. Fold cheese into mixture. While mixing, bake the pie crust for 10 minutes at 350° F. Pour mix into pie crust and bake one hour at 350° F or until it does not move when jiggled. Serve in wedges. Packages easily in plastic wrap.

### SERVE WITH:

Melon wedges

Crunchy granola w/carob chips, which is good by itself or on top of yogurt

Lemonade

**SUPER FOOD**

**Spinach** contains calcium, folic acid, magnesium, potassium, riboflavin (vitamin B2), and vitamins C and K. Spinach also contains lutein, which has been linked to lowering levels of artery-clogging fat deposits. Add in spinach, kale, collard greens, and other dark leafy green vegetables to your diet—use a few leaves of spinach instead of iceberg lettuce for sandwiches, for example, or chop up spinach leaves and add them to spaghetti sauce. Lightly cooked spinach is a delicacy, and it can be eaten raw as a salad green.

## SPAGHETTI PIE

1 16-ounce box spinach spaghetti
2 tablespoons extra virgin olive oil
1/3 cup grated parmesan
3 eggs, beaten
1 pound extra lean ground beef or turkey
1 jar spaghetti sauce
1/2 cup shredded mozzarella cheese
1 cup cottage cheese

Cook spaghetti as directed, then drain and stir in oil, parmesan cheese, and eggs. Form into a crust in the bottom of a greased 10" pie plate. Spread cottage cheese over spaghetti mixture. In skillet, cook meat, drain, and add sauce. Stir and heat thoroughly. Pour evenly over cottage cheese. Bake at 350° F for 20 minutes. Sprinkle mozzarella on top and bake until cheese melts.

This is an excellent meal to prepare for the family and send leftovers in school lunches. Or you can prepare and freeze in individual servings and take out as needed.

### SERVE WITH:

Diced apple and banana with 2 tablespoons of strawberry yogurt

Passion fruit dessert

Sparkling water with lime wedge

**SUPER FOOD**

**Eggs** are nearly a perfect food. The protein is complete, with all the essential amino acids, and the ratio of minerals is perfect for the purpose of growth. They contain high amounts of vitamins A, D, and E as well as some B-vitamins. Because egg yolks contain fat and cholesterol, many people think they should avoid them, but cholesterol is required by the body to make hormones, including the stress-fighting steroid hormones. Also, they contain rich amounts of lecithin, which prevents cholesterol from working much of its trouble in the arteries.

## SALMON QUESADILLAS

2 garlic cloves
Extra virgin olive oil
1 15-ounce can salmon, drained, boned, and skinned
2 tablespoons chopped cilantro
1/2 teaspoon pepper
2 cups shredded mozzarella cheese
1/2 cup corn
1/2 cup black beans
4 tablespoons softened butter
1/2 teaspoon sea salt
6 whole grain tortillas

In skillet, sauté garlic in extra virgin olive oil until tender. Stir in salmon, cilantro, salt, pepper, corn, and beans. Heat through about 10 minutes. Spread butter on 1 side of each tortilla. Heat separate skillet and warm tortilla butter-side down, sprinkling 1/2 cup cheese and 1/2 cup salmon mixture on one half of tortilla. Fold over and cook on low for 1 to 2 minutes on each side. Let cool 5 to 10 minutes and cut into wedges.

### SERVE WITH:

Guacamole
All natural corn chips
Watermelon wedge
Natural limeade

**SUPER FOOD**

**Salmon** is a marine and freshwater fish of the Northern Hemisphere that is a rich source of the Omega-3 oils, which are very important to optimal brain function. Put salmon together with carrots, broccoli, and spinach, and you'll give the brain a super boost. The Pacific salmon—pink, sockeye, chinook, dog, silver, and masu—hatches, spawn, and dies in freshwater, but spends its adult life in the ocean. The Atlantic salmon is actually an ocean-run trout. A marine fish, it spawns in rivers on both sides of the Atlantic and then returns to the sea. It does not die after spawning as the Pacific salmon.

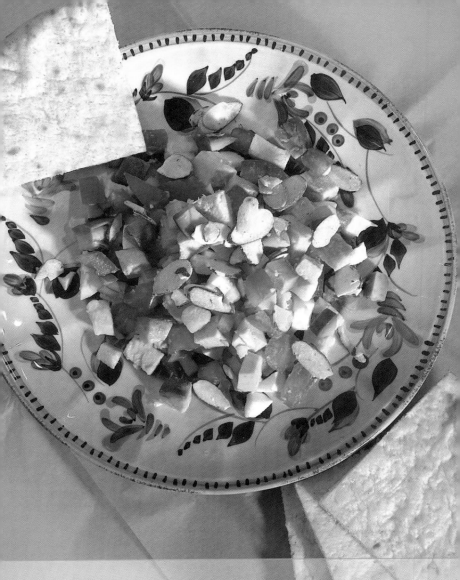

## TURKEY SALAD

2 cups cooked turkey, cut into 1/2" cubes
1/2 cup medium avocados (cut into 1/2" cubes)
1 ripe small tomato, seeded and diced (about 1/2 cup)
2 tablespoons diced red onions
1/4 cup slivered almonds
3 eggs, boiled and diced

Mix ingredients together.

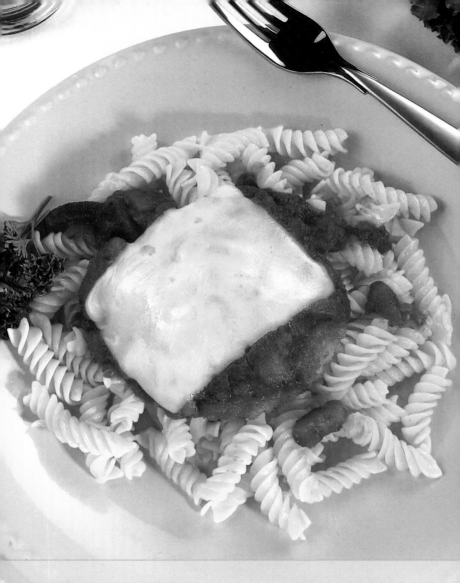

## FAUX CHICKEN PARMESAN

1 box vegetarian chicken patties
1 jar spaghetti sauce
Optional—pasta

Sliced mozzarella cheese
Optional—whole grain buns

Vegetarian chicken patties are found in the freezer section at the grocery store. Heat patties as directed. Heat sauce in small sauce pan. If serving with pasta, prepare pasta as directed. Combine pasta and chicken on a plate and cover with sauce. Top with cheese and heat under broiler until melted. With bun, prepare chicken and sauce the same and heat under broiler and serve.

## TURKEY BURGER

| | |
|---|---|
| 1–2 pounds ground turkey breast | 1/2 cup bread crumbs |
| 1/2 cup finely chopped onion | Sea salt |
| 3 eggs | Extra virgin olive oil |
| Whole grain buns | |

Combine all ingredients except oil. Pour small amount of oil in skillet. Shape mix into patties and cook through on each side. For those who like a little spice, such as my seven-year-old, Zachary, add a 1/4 cup salsa to mix. Make extra and freeze in individual baggies and take out as needed.

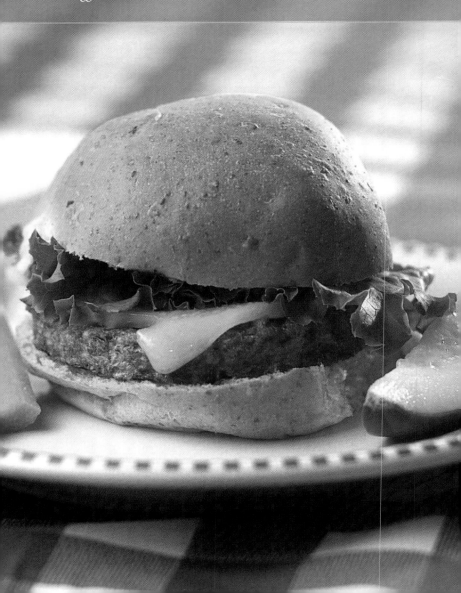

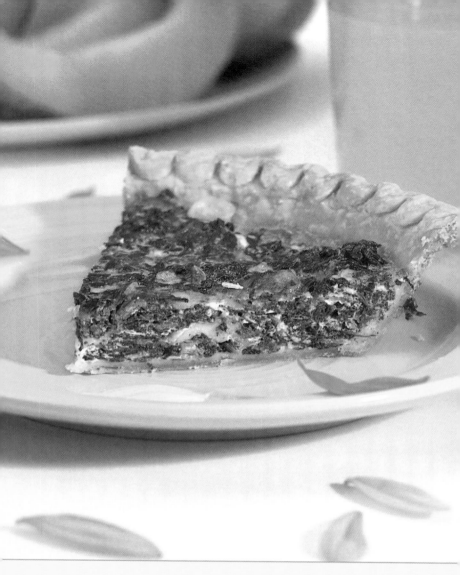

## SPINACH QUICHE

1 8-ounce package frozen spinach, cooked and drained
1/4 cup chopped onion        3–4 tablespoons extra virgin olive oil
1/4 teaspoon nutmeg          1 9" deep dish frozen pie crust
3 eggs, beaten               1/2 cup milk
1 1/2 cup shredded Swiss cheese    Sea salt to taste

Sauté onions in extra virgin olive oil and add in beaten eggs and milk. Add cooked spinach, nutmeg, and salt. Mix thoroughly. Fold cheese into mixture. While mixing, bake the pie crust for 10 minutes at 350° F. Pour mix into pie crust and bake one hour at 350° F or until it does not move when jiggled. Serve in wedges. Packages easily in plastic wrap.

## SALMON PATTIES

1 15-ounce can salmon, drained, boned, and skinned
3 eggs, beaten
1/2 cup bread crumbs
1/4 onion, diced
1 teaspoon dill weed
Sea salt to taste
Extra virgin olive oil

Drain salmon and remove skin and larger bones. I leave the small bones for added calcium. Combine salmon, eggs, onions, bread crumbs, dill weed, and salt together and mix thoroughly. Heat extra virgin olive oil over medium heat. Form patties and cook until brown on each side and solid.

These are great served hot or cold. My kids love them so much they even eat them for breakfast. I always make extra for a healthy snack by simply doubling or tripling the ingredients. Nice with ranch dressing on the side.

### SERVE WITH:

Avocado wedges (also nice to dip in ranch dressing)
Banana, apple yogurt salad
Carob chip and walnut cookie
Lemonade

**SUPER FOOD**

**Extra virgin olive oil** is by far the best oil you can use. It has been proven to be the healthiest for your heart as well as lowering your cholesterol level instead of clogging your arteries the way the saturated fats found in your typical grocery store oils and margarinated butter does. Stay away from Canola oil as well. Olive oil is far more versatile and can be used for just about anything. Medicinally speaking, olive oil has proven to be a natural antibiotic as well as antiviral. It tastes great and is good for you!

## BANANA FLAN PIE

3 freckled bananas
3 eggs
2 cups plain yogurt
1 tablespoon favorite jam/jelly
1 graham cracker crust

In blender, mix bananas, eggs, yogurt, and jam until smooth. Pour into crust and bake for one hour or until firm at 350° F.

This is one of my kids' favorite desserts . . . and everyone who's tried it at our house. It is so easy! I also throw in those little leftovers in the refrigerator for extra flavor—a couple of berries, a dab of cream cheese or cottage cheese, the partial cup of flavored yogurt leftovers, and more. Get creative!

## YOGURT PIE

1 cup plain organic yogurt
1 8-ounce package cream cheese softened
2 tablespoons honey
1 teaspoon vanilla
1 8"-graham cracker pie crust
2 cups pitted prunes halved, or apricots, strawberries, blueberries, etc.

With mixer or wooden spoon, beat yogurt, cream cheese, honey, and vanilla until smooth. Pour half into the crust. Top with an even layer of fruit. Cover with balance of yogurt mix. Refrigerate for 6 hours or until firm.

## YOGURT PARFAIT

1 quart vanilla yogurt
1 cup homemade granola
2 cups fresh berries
4–6 parfait cups or plastic storage bowl to go

Start with yogurt, then fruit, then granola, making two layers of each. Great as an afternoon snack or with lunch.

## COCOA COCONUT MACAROONS

2 egg whites
2/3 cup fructose
2 teaspoons vanilla
dash of sea salt
1 1/2 cups unsweetened coconut
2 tablespoons cocoa

Preheat oven to 300° F. Beat egg whites in a glass bowl until foamy. Add fructose a little at a time and continue beating until egg whites are stiff but not dry. Stir in vanilla, salt, and cocoa. Fold in coconut and stir gently. Drop by teaspoonful onto a lightly greased cookie sheet. Bake at 300° F for 15 minutes or until lightly browned. Cool for 5 minutes and remove.

## ANN'S GRANOLA BARS

1/2 cup honey
1/2 cup water
1/2 cup extra virgin olive oil
2 large eggs
2 tablespoons molasses
2 cups organic oats
1 1/2 cup whole wheat or spelt flour
2 teaspoons cinnamon
1 teaspoon baking powder
1/4–1/2 teaspoon sea salt

Preheat oven to 350° F. Mix ingredients but don't over stir. Butter and flour a 9" x 13" glass baking dish. Pour in mixture—should be somewhat soft. Bake at 350° F for 18 to 22 minutes. Do not over bake. Cool and slice. Ready to eat or wrap individually for school lunches.

Optional: Add sunflower seeds or organic raisins. Add 1/2 cup water or 1 freckled banana mashed or 1/3 cup sifted carob powder.

## LIVE TO 120 BIRTHDAY CAKE

1 cup real butter
1 1/2 cups honey
4 eggs beaten
2 cups sifted flour or wheat spelt
2 teaspoons baking soda
1 teaspoon ground cinnamon
1 teaspoon ground ginger
1/4 teaspoon sea salt
1 1/3 cup sour cream or plain yogurt

Preheat oven to 325° F. Cream together honey and butter. Add eggs. Add dry ingredients alternately with sour cream. Bake in two oiled and floured 9" cake pans at 325° F for 35 to 40 minutes. Ice cooled cake with cream cheese frosting.

## CREAM CHEESE FROSTING

8 ounces cream cheese
1/2 cup soft butter
1/4 cup honey
1/2 teaspoon vanilla

## BUGS ON A BOAT

Celery slices
Almond butter
Organic raisins
Banana slices

Put almond butter on celery slices and line raisins down the center. Use the bananas as your boat sail.

## CAROB BROWNIES

3 eggs
1/3 cup honey
1/4 cup extra virgin olive oil
2 teaspoons vanilla
2 freckled bananas
1/2 teaspoon sea salt
1 teaspoon baking powder
1/3 cup bottled water
1/3 cup sifted carob powder
1 cup whole wheat or spelt flour
1 cup chopped walnuts

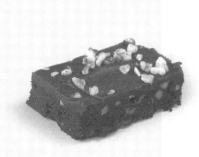

Preheat oven to 350° F. Beat eggs slightly, then add honey, oil, vanilla, and bananas. Mix well. Add dry ingredients alternately with water. Fold in walnuts. Butter and flour a 9" x 13" glass baking dish. Bake 23 minutes at 350° F. Do not over bake. If desired, top with brownie icing when warm. Cool before cutting.

## OPTIONAL BROWNIE ICING

4 tablespoons melted butter
2 teaspoons vanilla
1/3 cup honey
1/4 cup sifted carob powder

Mix all ingredients until smooth. Ice brownies.

## MINERAL TONIC

4–6 ounces organic milk or rice milk
1 tablespoon unsulfured blackstrap molasses

If you or your child are weak or anemic, this is an excellent drink to make as part of your daily routine.

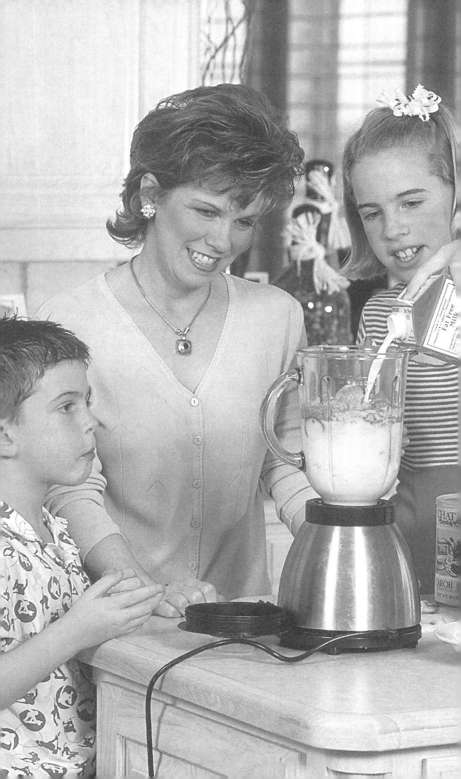

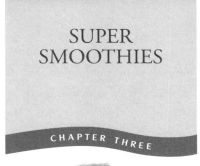

# SUPER SMOOTHIES

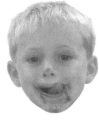

## CHAPTER THREE

SMOOTHIES ARE DELICIOUS, creamy health drinks made out of soft fruit. They make perfect energy boosters at any time of the day or can be used as a quick and easy substitute for meals. With the right ingredients, they are low in fat and high in essential nutrients. With a high-speed blender these can be made easily in five minutes and are quite filling and satisfying. Use your favorite fruits and juices in any combination you like to make a limitless variety of healthy drinks. A frozen smoothie makes for a mouth-watering dessert.

If you struggle to get your child to eat the recommended portions of five fruits and vegetables per day, smoothies are the way to go. Kids love to help create the drinks and watch the blender work. Toss in a frozen banana or ice cubes to chill the smoothie and give it a refreshing quality. Smoothies also allow you to add in powdered or liquid supplements as well as seeds that deliver rich nutrients.

Several of the smoothie recipes include *Creation's Bounty*, which is simply the best, pleasant tasting, green, whole raw organic food supplement. A blend of whole, raw organic herbs and grains—principally amaranth, brown rice, spirulina, and flaxseed—this combination of live foods provides your family with vital nutrients, living enzymes, and extra energy. *Brain Sharpener* is an herbal and natural combination shown to bring cognitive improvement, mental clarity, concentration, and creativity, enhancing optimum brainpower for your kids. Both *Creation's Bounty* and *Brain Sharpener* are available through Silver Creek Labs, which can be found on page 123.

### Mom's Favorite
1 cup ice
1 1/2 cup organic milk or rice milk
2 organic bananas
8 strawberries
2 heaping scoops of Creation's Bounty
1 cup plain yogurt

Fill balance of blender with distilled water
Blend and enjoy.

### Everything's Peachy
1 cup ice
1 cup rice milk
1 serving Spirutein Peach Smoothie
2 scoops Creation's Bounty
1 cup organic peach yogurt

Fill balance of blender with distilled water
Blend thoroughly.

### Dad's Berry Berry Smoothie
1 cup ice
1 cup vanilla yogurt
1/2 cup strawberries
1/2 cup blueberries
1/2 cup raspberries
1 cup mango kerns juice

Fill balance of blender with distilled water
Blend until smooth.

## Make Believe Reese's Cup Smoothie
1 cup ice
1 organic banana
2 tablespoons honey
1 tablespoon carob powder
2 tablespoons almond butter
2 scoops Creation's Bounty
1 cup yogurt
1 cup rice or organic milk

Fill balance of blender with distilled water
Blend and enjoy.

## Morgan's (age 11) Tropical Delight Smoothie
1 cup ice
1 cup organic strawberry yogurt
1 cup rice milk
1 cup fresh pineapple cut in cubes
2 organic bananas
1 tablespoon Hawaiian Spirulina
6–8 fresh strawberries
2 scoops Creation's Bounty

Fill balance of blender with distilled water
Blend until smooth.

## Lexie's (age 16) Coffee-Loving Smoothie
1 cup ice
1 cup distilled water
1 cup organic milk
2 scoops Capacino Spirutein Smoothie Mix
2 scoops Creation's Bounty
1 cup organic coffee yogurt

Blend.

## Whitney's (age 18) Energy Smoothie
1 cup ice
1 cup apple juice
1 tablespoon Hawaiian Spirulina
1 teaspoon local bee pollen
1 tablespoon local honey
2 scoops Creation's Bounty
1 organic banana
1 cup vanilla yogurt

Fill balance of blender with distilled water
Blend.

## Cortney's (age 22) Everything But the Kitchen Sink Smoothie
1 cup ice
1-ounce liquid minerals
1 scoop Creation's Bounty
1 scoop fiber supplement
1 scoop vanilla protein powder
1 teaspoon calcium magnesium
2000 mg. vitamin C
1 large organic banana
1 cup yogurt
1 cup frozen berries
1 1/2 cup Juicy Juice

Blend.

## Zach (age 7) Attack Smoothie
1 cup ice
2 frozen organic bananas
2 scoops chocolate protein powder
1 scoop Creation's Bounty
1 cup plain yogurt
1 cup organic milk

Fill balance of blender with distilled water
Blend.

## Hamilton's (age 15) Ham the Muscle Man Smoothie
1 cup ice
1 cup plain yogurt
1 cup organic milk
2 scoops vanilla protein powder
2 scoops Creation's Bounty
1 tablespoon vanilla extract
2 organic bananas
1 teaspoon nutmeg

Blend.

## Seth's (almost 1, but he knows what's good) Funny Bunny Smoothie
1 cup ice
1 cup fresh carrot juice
1 cup plain yogurt
1 teaspoon bee pollen
2 scoops Creation's Bounty
1 organic banana
3-ounces tofu
1 teaspoon Spirulina

Fill balance of blender with distilled water
Blend.

## Jesse's (age 10) Zany Brainy Smoothie
1 cup ice
1 1/2 cup apple juice
1 cup yogurt
1 organic banana
6 fresh strawberries
1/2 cup frozen peaches
1-ounce flaxseed oil
3 Brain Sharpeners punctured and drained into mix
2 scoops Creation's Bounty

Fill balance of blender with distilled water
Blend.

## Smooth Moves Smoothie
1 cup ice
1 cup prune juice
1 tablespoon blackstrap molasses
1 cup organic milk
1 cup plain yogurt
1 organic banana
2 scoops Creation's Bounty
1 serving fiber

Fill balance of blender with distilled water
Blend.

## Pink Zinger Smoothie
2 freckled bananas
1/2 cup fresh strawberries
2 cups pink grapefruit juice, unsweetened
1 cup ice

Blend and serve.

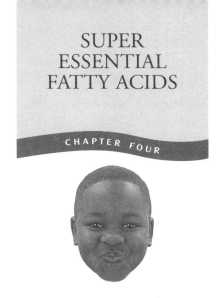

# SUPER ESSENTIAL FATTY ACIDS

## CHAPTER FOUR

FAT IS AS ESSENTIAL TO OUR DIETS as any other component, despite the constant warnings we have heard about it. Fat helps to build cell membranes in every cell in the body. Good fats, essential fatty acids, affect the brain so much that every area of sensory and motor skills either improves or declines through what you eat. These fats ensure that the nervous system functions properly. Sixty-five percent of the brain is made up of good fats, and we must have these good fats for proper brain function and increased memory. Children can develop ADD or ADHD at a very early age because of the lack of essential fatty acids combined with the increased sugars that are in the foods we give our children.

While it's true that we eat far too many saturated (usually hard or solid at room temperature) and hydrogenated fats from sources such as meat, dairy products, margarine, cooking oils, and packaged food, certain fats are needed for good health. Unsaturated fats (usually soft at room temperature and often called oils) are divided into monounsaturated fats and polyunsaturated fats.

Monounsaturated fats appear to provide some protection from heart disease and are the best for cooking, as they do not tend to undergo chemical changes when they are heated. Polyunsaturated fats are prone to changes when they are exposed to light, heat, the air, and other chemicals. If they are processed, such as in the manufacture of margarine, chemical changes can occur, leading to the production of "trans-fats." These are fats that the body cannot easily break down and often lead to blocked arteries and heart disease. Trans-fatty acids are contained in foods such as ice cream, potato chips, tortilla chips, burgers, chicken nuggets, French fries, fried foods, candy, cookies, cakes, donuts, margarine, shortening, mayonnaise, partially hydrogenated oils, puffed cheese snacks, and dressing—which happens to be on the menu for many Americans on a regular basis.

Two polyunsaturated fatty acids, linoleic acid and alpha-linolenic acid, are known as essential fatty acids because our body does not produce them. These come mainly from the Omega family of fats. Good Omega-3 fats include: flaxseed, hemp seed, pumpkin seed, soy, wheat germ, walnuts, leafy green vegetables, borage seed oil, fish oil, salmon, trout, mackerel, herring, blue fin, sardines, anchovies, and white albacore tuna. Good Omega-6 fats include: walleye, carp, pike, haddock, sesame oil, borage seed oil, evening primrose oil, unrefined sunflower oil, walnuts, chicken, rice bran, black current seeds, fresh unroasted and unsalted nuts and seeds, and eggs. Good Omega-9 fats include: extra virgin olive oil, avocados, and meats.

If you go on a low-fat diet, be sure you are working with a counselor to ensure you are getting enough unsaturated fatty acids and a balance of the Omega oils. For optimal behavior and mood function, there must be a balance. Dr. Michael Schmidt, an Applied Biochemistry and Clinical Nutritionist at Northwestern College, has shown that an imbalance contributes to depression, postpartum depression, OCD, problems with MS patients, winter blues, fears and phobias, chronic fatigue, attention problems, hyperactivity, violence and aggression, schizophrenia, stress response, mood swings, and behavioral problems. He also noted that cultures that eat lots of fish (high in Omega 3 and 6) show little to no depression problems.

Dr. E. A. Mitchell and his colleagues studied ADD and ADHD in children. They found continually low levels of Omega 3 and 6—the two key brain fats. Hyperactive children were shown to have higher levels of Omega 6 and lower levels of Omega 3. When Omega 6 is higher than Omega 3, there is lower brain function. He also showed that breast-fed children are less likely to have ADHD due to high contents of essential fatty acids in the milk.

**Cheat Sheet:** Good fats help every function in the body, especially the brain, and are God-made—nuts, avocados, fish, olive oil, etc. Bad fats bring harm and are man-made—marjoram, ice cream, processed cheese, fried foods, etc.

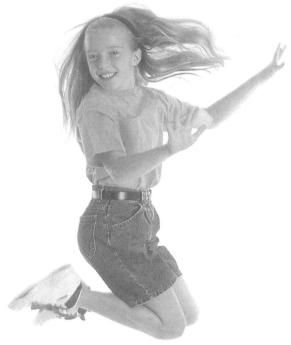

# SUPER COMPLEX CARBOHYDRATES

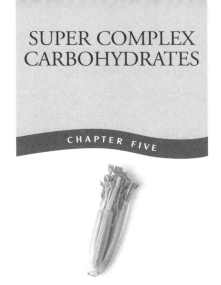

## CHAPTER FIVE

COMPLEX CARBOHYDRATES ARE DERIVED from carbon, hydrogen, and oxygen. Sugar, starch, and cellulose are carbohydrates. They are a major source of energy in our diet and are found in grains, legumes, fruits, vegetables, sugar, and alcohol. They have beneficial effects on the way we absorb and use our nutrients. During the digestion of food, carbohydrates in the food are broken down into smaller sugar molecules such as fructose, galactose, and glucose. These are the body and the brain's favorite fuel because it helps to maintain concentration, keeps us mentally sharp, and provides the power for all the brain's functions. Children need sufficient levels of carbohydrates not only because they are so active but because they need energy to grow.

You need to keep in mind that some carbohydrates release their energy slowly and provide long-lasting sustenance to the body and the brain. These are the ones you want—primarily the brown grains and rice, fruits, or leafy green foods with all their fiber intact. One value of the fiber is that it prolongs the carbohydrate's energy release for hours after you've eaten. These foods are more "complex" than simple carbohydrates.

Then there are the simple carbohydrates that release

quickly—the refined white starchy foods, sugars, and alcohol. They deliver a burst of energy by the quick breakdown into glucose and release into the bloodstream, but they leave you soon exhausted and unable to concentrate. The effects of a drop in blood sugar levels can also include nervousness, hyperactivity, confusion, depression, anxiety, forgetfulness, headaches, palpitations, dizziness, and insomnia.

Researchers have also discovered that the constant insulin "highs" produced by fluctuating blood sugar levels lead to an increase in body weight. Insulin stimulates an enzyme called lipoprotein-lipase, which directs circulating fatty acids into fat-cell storage, which increase body weight. Children who are allowed to snack on cookies, ice cream, candy, cakes, and potato chips will put on the weight.

Sugar is the most addictive substance in our diets, and food manufacturers know it. You'll find sugar in almost every processed or packaged food, and the cumulative effect is reflected in bulging waistlines and poor health. You have to cut out the heavy intake of sugar.

Excellent carbohydrate sources are vegetables of all kinds (raw whenever possible), fruits, legumes, milk, whole grains, and whole wheat pasta. The good news is that foods containing complex carbohydrates, such as bread and pasta, are usually rich in vitamins, minerals, and trace elements.

**Cheat Sheet:** Good carbs are essential! Foods such as fresh fruit and veggies, brown rice, oats, and beans provide good, slow-burning energy. Bad carbs such as processed sugary snacks, chips, breads, muffins, and candy pick you up quickly and drop you like a lead balloon.

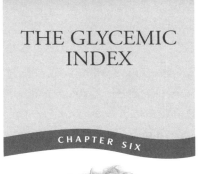

# THE GLYCEMIC INDEX

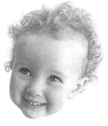

## CHAPTER SIX

As mentioned previously, complex carbohydrates burn more slowly and, for the most part, help regulate the amount of sugar released into the bloodstream. The rate at which blood sugar levels rise after a specific food is eaten is called its glycemic index, which was devised as a means to help diabetics in their food selections. One of the values of this general index is that it shows that even among carbohydrates, there is a wide range of variance of values. For instance, the potato is actually a high-glycemic food that can spike one's insulin levels and should be eaten in moderation.

The numbers below are based on glucose, which is the fastest carbohydrate available except for maltose. *Glucose is given a value of 100—other carbs are given a number relative to glucose.* Any glycemic value over 50 (other experts say 60) is considered to be high (that's one-half the value of glucose). Faster carbs (higher numbers) are great for raising low blood sugars and for covering brief periods of intense exercise. Slower carbs (lower numbers) are helpful for preventing overnight drops in the blood sugar and for long periods of exercise.

These numbers are compiled from a wide range of research labs, and as often as possible from more than one study. These numbers will be close but may not be identical to other glycemic index lists. The impact a food will have on blood sugars depends on many other factors like ripeness, cooking time, fiber and fat content, time of day, blood insulin levels, and recent activity. Use the Glycemic Index as just one of the many tools you have available to improve your control.

## Beans
baby lima . . . . . . .32
baked . . . . . . . . . .43
black . . . . . . . . . .30
brown . . . . . . . . . .38
butter . . . . . . . . . .31
chickpeas . . . . . . .33
kidney . . . . . . . . .27
lentil . . . . . . . . . . .30
navy . . . . . . . . . . .38
pinto . . . . . . . . . . .42
red lentils . . . . . . .27
split peas . . . . . . .32
soy . . . . . . . . . . . .18

## Breads
bagel . . . . . . . . . .72
croissant . . . . . . . .67
Kaiser roll . . . . . . .73
pita . . . . . . . . . . .57
pumpernickel . . . .49
rye . . . . . . . . . . . .64
rye, dark . . . . . . .76
rye, whole . . . . . . .50
white . . . . . . . . . .72
whole wheat . . . . .72

## Cereals
All Bran . . . . . . . .44
Bran Chex . . . . . . .58
Cheerios . . . . . . . .74
Corn Bran . . . . . . .75
Corn Chex . . . . . .83
Cornflakes . . . . . .83
Cream of Wheat . .66
Crispix . . . . . . . . .87

Frosted Flakes . . . .55
Grapenuts . . . . . . .67
Grapenuts Flakes . .80
Life . . . . . . . . . . . .66
Muesli . . . . . . . . . .60
NutriGrain . . . . . .66
Oatmeal . . . . . . . .49
Oatmeal 1 min . . .66
Puffed Wheat . . . .74
Puffed Rice . . . . . .90
Rice Bran . . . . . . .19
Rice Chex . . . . . . .89
Rice Krispies . . . . .82
Shredded Wheat . .69
Special K . . . . . . .54
Swiss Muesli . . . . .60
Total . . . . . . . . . . .76

## Cookies
Graham crackers . . .74
oatmeal . . . . . . . .55
shortbread . . . . . .64
Vanilla Wafers . . .77

## Crackers
rice cakes . . . . . . .82
rye . . . . . . . . . . . .63
saltine . . . . . . . . . .72
stoned wheat thins . .67
water crackers . . . .78

## Desserts
angel food cake . .67
banana bread . . . .47
blueberry muffin . .59

bran muffin . . . . . .60
Danish . . . . . . . . .59
fruit bread . . . . . . .47
pound cake . . . . . .54
sponge cake . . . . .46

## Fruit
apple . . . . . . . . . .38
apricot, canned . . .64
apricot, dried . . . .30
banana . . . . . . . . .62
banana, unripe . . .30
cantaloupe . . . . . .65
cherries . . . . . . . . .22
dates, dried . . . . .103
fruit cocktail . . . . .55
grapefruit . . . . . . .25
grapes . . . . . . . . .43
kiwi . . . . . . . . . . .52
mango . . . . . . . . .55
orange . . . . . . . . .43
papaya . . . . . . . . .58
peach . . . . . . . . . .42
pear . . . . . . . . . . .36
pineapple . . . . . . .66
plum . . . . . . . . . . .24
raisins . . . . . . . . . .64
strawberries . . . . .32
strawberry jam . . .51
watermelon . . . . . .72

## Grains
barley . . . . . . . . . .22
brown rice . . . . . .59
buckwheat . . . . . .54

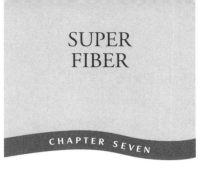

# SUPER FIBER

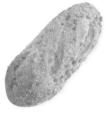

## CHAPTER SEVEN

FIBER COMES FROM THE CELLS WALLS and other parts of plants, with fresh, live foods being the best source. It is a key to a low glycemic diet and essential for good health. A diet rich in fiber can help fight obesity, heart disease, diabetes, and cancer. It slows down the digestive process and helps regulate the release of insulin into the bloodstream, which allows for a steady supply of energy over a longer period of time. Beyond that, fiber speeds the transit time of fecal matter out of the body, which makes it highly valuable.

While Americans eat an average of 12–17 grams of fiber daily, the American Dietetic Association recommends an intake of 20–25 grams, and some experts say that for optimal health a person should get 40–60 grams a day.

Fiber comes in two forms: soluble and insoluble. Soluble fiber, which is present in legumes, brans, fruits, vegetable, whole grain products, seeds and nuts, and psyllium seed, helps to reduce cholesterol and balance blood sugar levels. Insoluble fiber, found in whole wheat products, brown rice, kidney beans, skins of fruits, and many vegetables, reduce the risk of constipation as well as help prevent bowel cancer.

**Cheat Sheet:** Good fiber is found in a bowl of oat bran and fresh fruit. A pathetic attempt is a bran muffin loaded with processed sugars and preservatives.

## A Sample of Fiber Content of Foods
(fiber value is in grams)

Almonds (slivered, dried, 1 cup) . . . . . . . . . . . . . . . . . .14.7
Apple (small, with skin) . . . . . . . . . . . . . . . . . . . . . . . .3.0
Avocado (1 whole) . . . . . . . . . . . . . . . . . . . . . . . . . . .4.7
Bacon . . . . . . . . . . . . . . . . . . . . . . . . . . . . . . . . . . . .0
Beans, kidney (1/2 cup) . . . . . . . . . . . . . . . . . . . . . .10.0
Beans, sprouts (1/2 cup) . . . . . . . . . . . . . . . . . . . . . .8.2
Bran, oat (1/2 cup) . . . . . . . . . . . . . . . . . . . . . . . . .10.5
Bran, wheat (1/2 cup) . . . . . . . . . . . . . . . . . . . . . . .15.6
Carrots (chopped, 1/2 cup) . . . . . . . . . . . . . . . . . . .2.78
Cornmeal (stone ground, 1/2 cup) . . . . . . . . . . . . . . .6.0
Doughnuts . . . . . . . . . . . . . . . . . . . . . . . . . . . . . . . . .0
Figs (dried, chopped, 1/2 cup) . . . . . . . . . . . . . . . . . .7.5
Flour, all-purpose white (1 cup) . . . . . . . . . . . . . . . . . .3.4
Flour, whole wheat (1 cup) . . . . . . . . . . . . . . . . . . . .13.0
Lentils (cooked, 1/2 cup) . . . . . . . . . . . . . . . . . . . . . .7.8
Lettuce, romaine (shredded, 1/2 cup) . . . . . . . . . . . . .0.7
Meat . . . . . . . . . . . . . . . . . . . . . . . . . . . . . . . . . . . . .0
Pasta, whole wheat (1 cup) . . . . . . . . . . . . . . . . . . . .6.3
Pear (1 medium) . . . . . . . . . . . . . . . . . . . . . . . . . . . .4.6
Pepper, green (1 large) . . . . . . . . . . . . . . . . . . . . . . .0.9
Potato, white (2.25" diameter) . . . . . . . . . . . . . . . . . .2.1
Prunes, dried (8 large) . . . . . . . . . . . . . . . . . . . . . . .16.1
Raisins (1/2 cup) . . . . . . . . . . . . . . . . . . . . . . . . . . . .5.4
Raspberries (1/2 cup) . . . . . . . . . . . . . . . . . . . . . . . .6.4
Rice, Brown (1/2 cup) . . . . . . . . . . . . . . . . . . . . . . . .4.2
Soybeans (1/2 cup) . . . . . . . . . . . . . . . . . . . . . . . . . .9.6
Spaghetti, white (1/2 cup) . . . . . . . . . . . . . . . . . . . .0.15
Strawberries (1/2 cup) . . . . . . . . . . . . . . . . . . . . . . . .1.7

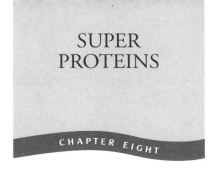

# SUPER
# PROTEINS

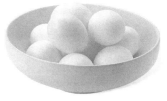

## CHAPTER EIGHT

**AS THE FAMED BUILDING BLOCKS** of the body, proteins consist of long, folded chains of amino acids. Protein is one of the three main classes of nutrients that provide energy to the body (the others are carbohydrates and fats), and I highlight them because of their importance in regard to nutrition. You need them for building and repairing body tissues, and for producing hormones, enzymes, and nerve chemicals. Proteins exist in every cell and are essential to life. They are vital for sustaining a healthy immune system and to building the brain's messengers—the neurotransmitters. And they need to be taken in daily, because your body cannot store them. We must obtain most of them from the foods we eat.

Proteins are large, complex molecules made up of small units called amino acids. The amino acids are linked together into long chains called polypeptides. Twenty amino acids are assembled into the thousands of different proteins required by the human body. To assemble the proteins it needs, the body must have a sufficient supply of all these amino acids. Some amino acids, called essential amino acids, cannot be produced by the body and must be supplied by various foods. Humans require nine essential amino acids, and for the body to use the amino acids properly, all these amino acids must be present at the same time and in the correct proportions. A shortage or absence of just one essential amino acid results in the body's not being able to make any of the other necessary amino acids. The remaining acids, called nonessential amino acids, can be manufactured by the body itself.

When protein is eaten, your digestive processes break it down into amino acids, which pass into the blood and are carried throughout the body. Your cells can then select the amino acids they need for the construction of tissue repair and new body tissue (especially bone cartilage and muscle), antibodies, hormones, enzymes, and worn-out and dead blood cells. Every cell needs protein to maintain its life.

Your muscles, hair, nails, skin, and eyes are made of protein. So are the cells that make up the liver, kidneys, heart, lungs, nerves, brain, and your sex glands. The body's most active protein users are the hormones secreted from the various glands—thyroxin from the thyroid, insulin from the pancreas, and a variety of hormones from the pituitary—as well as the soft tissues, hardworking major organs, and muscles. Two amino acids, tyrosine and tryptophan, are vital to making the two key neurotransmitters that regulate your child's mood and lift depression. They all require the richest stores of protein.

The complete proteins that contain the essential amino acids come from meat, poultry, fish, eggs, milk—all dairy products. These same foods are also high in saturated fats, which is not desirable. Cereal grains, nuts, legumes (peas and beans), and vegetables contain some but not all of the essential amino acids and can be used to ensure the adequate supply of the amino acids required to promote physical and mental health. For example, ounce for ounce, steak contains less protein than soy flour. If possible, stay away from foods that have been smoked, are high in fat, or that contain chemical preservatives (such as most sausages).

The body is not able to store protein, and if excessive amounts are being consumed, they will be converted into sugars and fats. The idea that it is less fattening to feed your child lots of protein instead of carbohydrates is wrong. A balanced diet is the only way to ensure that your child is getting all the nutrients they need.

Insufficient protein in the diet may cause a lack of energy, stunted growth, and lowered resistance to disease. If the body does not receive enough proteins from the food eaten, it uses proteins from the cells of the liver and muscle tissues. Continued use of such proteins by the body can permanently damage those tissues.

**Cheat Sheet:** Protein is one of the areas I watch the most! Without proper protein, you cannot repair body tissue, can't think right, and can't grow right! It's that simple. Eat lots of eggs, milk, fish, poultry, meat, and nuts. This does not mean swing through the drive thru and get a burger to get your protein. You don't know what you may be getting!

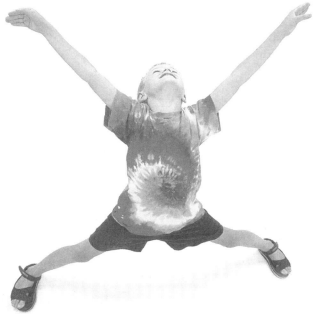

# SUPER ANTIOXIDANTS

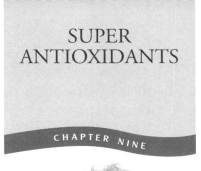

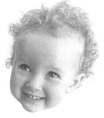

## CHAPTER NINE

IN THE PROCESS OF METABOLISM OR OXIDATION, our body cells produce molecules called free radicals. They are unstable molecules that attempt to steal electrons from any available source, such as our body tissues. Antioxidants, such as beta-carotene, vitamins A, E, and especially C, and selenium, work to neutralize these unstable chemicals and protect us from them. The more antioxidants we get in our diets, the more we are able to stop these damaging effects. The main source of antioxidants is fruits, vegetables, nuts, grains, and cold-pressed plant oils.

Antioxidants are essential for detoxification because they help cells neutralize free radicals that can cause mutations and cellular damage. This damage is partly responsible for a wide range of illnesses, including all the degenerative diseases such as arthritis, cardiovascular disease, Alzheimer's, and cancer. Any shortage of antioxidants can become catastrophic to one's health. When our antioxidants are low, energy is not available and detoxification cannot take place in a normal fashion. Therefore, toxins accumulate or are stored until they can be processed.

Other excellent sources of antioxidants are found in bioflavonoids, grape seed extract, ginseng, garlic, molybdenum,

DHEA, wheat and barley grass, Echinacea, manganese, carotenoids, Ginkgo Biloba, melatonin, L-Cysteine, acetyl-l-carnite, CoQ10, milk thistle, and B-vitamins.

**Cheat Sheet:** You must get your antioxidants! I supplement as well as make sure we eat the foods that contain them. Eat lots of God's foods, such as fresh fruits and veggies. Vitamin C and selenium are my favorite supplements.

# SUPER FISH

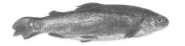

## CHAPTER TEN

ACCORDING TO LEVITICUS 11:9, fish is considered to be a clean food. Almost all fish are naturally low in calories and rich in health-giving oils as well as essential vitamins and minerals. Fish contain important Omega-3 fatty acids, which have been proven to lower cholesterol, inhibit blood clots, lower blood pressure, and reduce the risk of heart attack and stroke. Many fish are also delicious and quick-serving—a real convenience food.

For years cod liver oil has been used as an immune system booster and tonic to cure any number of ills. Today, medical experts are seeing the wisdom that has been in God's plan from the beginning of time. Researchers at Rutgers University have shown that fish oil is also an effective cancer fighter, reducing your risk of breast, pancreatic, lung, prostate, and colon cancers. Migraine sufferers also find great relief with Omega-3 fish oils, according to studies at the University of Cincinnati. Another study there showed that people who suffer from psoriasis were helped tremendously after taking Omega-3 fatty acid.

Shellfish and fish without scales are high in cholesterol and considered high-stress foods. Stay away from these. The best fish sources, which are naturally low in calories, are salmon, mackerel, and halibut.

To get the best fish, the freshest fish, look for a fish vendor with a high turnover. Make sure the whole fish is covered in ice. The fish eyes should be bright and clear, not sunken, and the skin should be shiny and unblemished. Fillets or steaks should have a moist, almost translucent sheen. Avoid any fish that has dried out or gaping flesh.

**Cheat Sheet:** If you don't like fish, *learn!* Fish provide nutrients and benefits for you that no other foods can. Jesus had fishermen on staff, which should tell us something. Fish are good brain and body food. Eat fish meals at least 2 to 3 times per week.

# YOGURT PARFAIT

1 quart vanilla yogurt
1 cup homemade granola
2 cups fresh berries
4–6 parfait cups or plastic storage bowl to go

Start with yogurt, then fruit, then granola, making two layers of each. Great as an afternoon snack or with lunch.

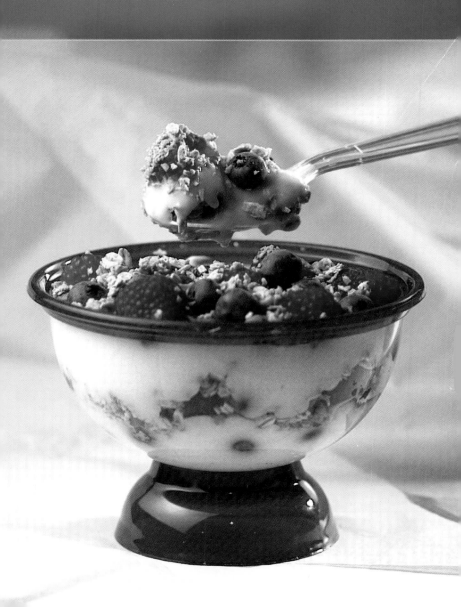

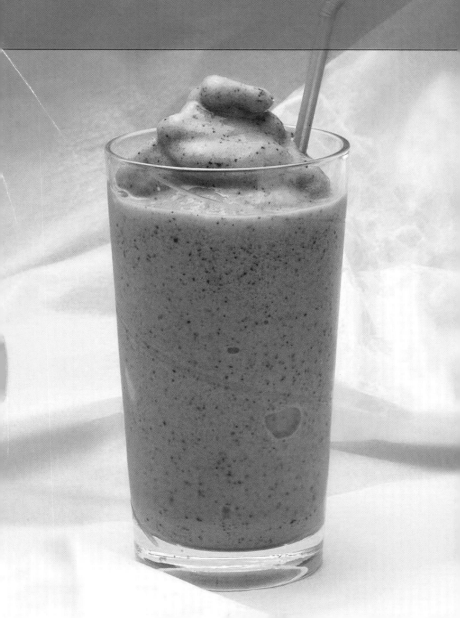

## DAD'S BERRY BERRY SMOOTHIE

| | |
|---|---|
| 1 cup ice | 1 cup vanilla yogurt |
| 1/2 cup strawberries | 1/2 cup blueberries |
| 1/2 cup raspberries | 1 cup mango kerns juice |

Fill balance of blender with distilled water. Blend until smooth.

## MORGAN'S (AGE 11) TROPICAL DELIGHT SMOOTHIE

1 cup ice
1 cup rice milk
2 organic bananas
6–8 fresh strawberries

1 cup organic strawberry yogurt
1 cup fresh pineapple cut in cubes
1 tablespoon Hawaiian Spirulina
2 scoops Creation's Bounty

Fill balance of blender with distilled water. Blend until smooth.

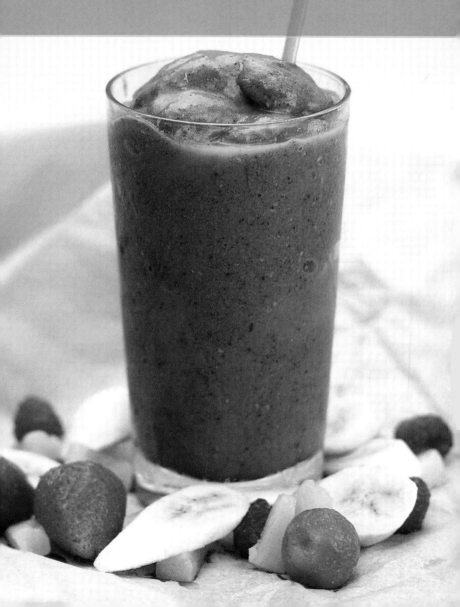

## QUICKIE PROTEIN SNACK OR BREAKFAST

1/2 cup organic cottage cheese (each serving is approximately
13–15 grams of protein)
Fresh pineapple cut in bite size or canned without syrup
A drizzle of real maple syrup

This is a tasty snack or quick breakfast that's high in protein. Everybody loves it!

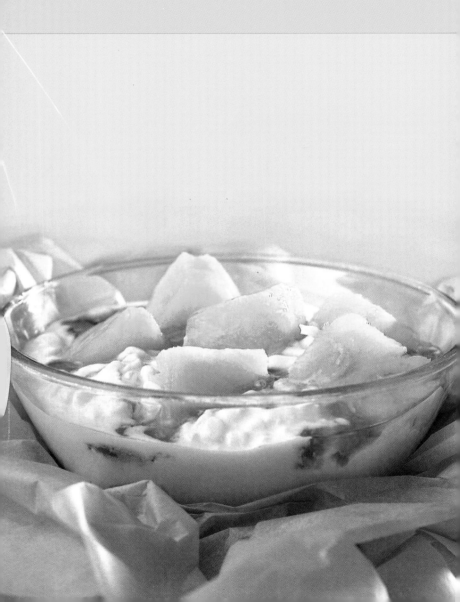

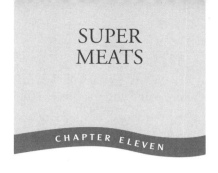

# SUPER MEATS

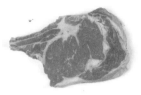

## CHAPTER ELEVEN

**CHICKEN HAS REPLACED BEEF** as America's favorite meat, and turkey is right behind. That's a healthy trend, since poultry is one of the leanest meats available, and it's a trend that you need to make sure is true in your family.

With poultry, the leanest meat is the breast, followed by the drumstick. The fattiest parts are the wings, which have a lot of skin and little meat, and the thighs. Always remove the skin to cut out the fat.

Whether it's a juicy hamburger or tender lamb chop, red meat holds a strong appeal among Americans. The fact remains that most of us need to cut down on our red meats because they are a primary source of saturated fat and cholesterol. It is true that meat producers are providing leaner beef and lamb. Always look for the lean cuts and keep your portions small. Trim off all the visible fat before cooking, and think 2–3 ounces as the serving size. I stay away from all pork meat because it is an unclean food, a non-Kosher food, according to biblical definitions.

Because of the crowded conditions and the antibiotics that are used routinely in most conventionally farmed poultry and live-stock, if at all possible buy free-range poultry and organic meats.

"Free range" ensures that the poultry was given a minimum of indoor and outdoor space. "Organic" means that the animal was raised outdoors, was fed organic food, and is free of antibiotics. I also highly recommend Kosher meats because their slaughtering methods are far more humane, which keeps hormones from being released in the animal's bloodstream and then spilling into the flesh.

**Cheat Sheet:** Chicken, turkey, and lamb are great with a little beef thrown in once a week. Go for the organic, hormone free meats . . . or stay away!

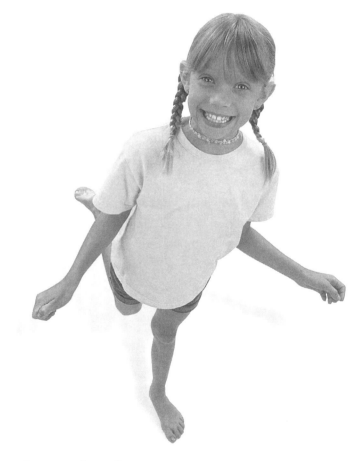

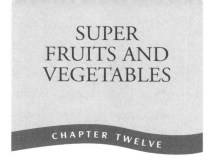

# SUPER FRUITS AND VEGETABLES

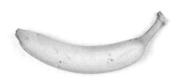

## CHAPTER TWELVE

**FRUITS AND VEGETABLES** are so packed with minerals, vitamins, chlorophyll, and enzymes that they're well worth turning into your main-dish meal rather than merely side dishes. These enzyme-rich foods make it possible to convert food into body tissue and the fuel to keep you going, and they are a must to keep you healthy. In addition, these foods contain phytochemicals or phytonutrients ("phyto" means "plant"). A single fruit or vegetable may contain several hundred phytochemicals, and many of these have been proven to promote health. Eating raw fruits and vegetables or juicing them delivers the full benefits to your system.

How you cook your vegetables will make a huge difference in preserving their nutrients and texture. Steam them or cook them in as small amount of water as possible, and you will preserve the water-soluble nutrients such as vitamin C. You can cut down the nutrient loss by not adding your vegetables until the water is boiling, thus reducing your cooking time. When the vegetable's color has intensified and they're tender-crisp, they are ready to eat.

With the prevalence of pesticides used on fruit and vegetable crops, which are designed to kill a variety of pests by damaging their brains and nerves, has come residue that interacts with the chemicals in our bodies. Because children are still growing, they are the most at risk from pesticide contamination, and some experts see a direct correlation between hyperactivity and pesticides.

Organically grown fruits and vegetables eliminate the concern over pesticides and have more vitamins and minerals than conventionally grown produce. Because organic farmers use natural fertilizers, which contain a wide variety of minerals that help maintain the balance of minerals in the soil, their fruit and vegetables contain more minerals such as calcium, iron, manganese, magnesium, and more protein and vitamins. They may be a bit more expensive, but they're well worth it.

Fruits and vegetables must always be washed thoroughly. Green leafy vegetables should be washed leaf by leaf. If your vegetables are not organic, root vegetables such as carrots and fruits such as apples and pears should always be peeled before eating or cooking because of the pesticides. It's always best to eat fresh fruits and vegetables, but convenience, season, and price may make that difficult. Keep frozen and canned goods on hand to make certain you're eating plenty of fruits and vegetables every day.

**Cheat Sheet:** Eat at least 5 servings per day—fresh, fresh, fresh! Organic, if possible. Remember: We started in the Garden of Eden. Hint . . . hint!

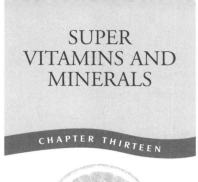

# SUPER VITAMINS AND MINERALS

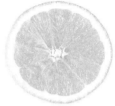

## CHAPTER THIRTEEN

VITAMINS CONSTITUTE ONE OF THE MAJOR GROUPS of nutrients, which are food substances necessary for growth and health. They regulate chemical reactions through which the body converts food into energy and living tissues. Thus they have a key role in producing energy for each and every cell in the body. Vitamins also help to manufacture enzymes, which do wide-ranging tasks within the body from digesting food to making neurotransmitters. Of the 13 vitamins we need, 5 are produced by the body itself. Of those 5, only 3 can be produced in sufficient quantities to meet the body's needs. Therefore, vitamins must be supplied in a person's daily diet.

We tend to think that any vitamin will do, but this is not the case. Every vitamin has a specific function that nothing else can replace. And, if you lack any vitamin, it can actually hinder the function of another. Vitamin deficiency diseases, such as beriberi, pellagra, rickets, or scurvy, are the result of an ongoing lack of a vitamin.

A well-balanced diet from all the basic food groups is the best way to obtain these essential vitamins. If you take supplements, always take a food-based multivitamin capsule as well as specific nutrients to help them work more effectively. Do not exceed the doses printed on the packaging.

Minerals are nutrients that function alongside vitamins as components of body enzymes. While they are needed in small amounts, they are absolutely essential for the biochemical processes of the body to work. Without your minerals in adequate supply, you can't absorb the vitamins. Minerals are needed for proper composition of teeth and bone and blood and muscle and nerve cells. They are important to the production of hormones and enzymes and in the creation of antibodies. Some minerals (calcium, potassium, and sodium) have electrical charges that act as a magnet to attract other electrically charged substances to form complex molecules, conduct electrical impulses (messages) along nerves, and transport substances in and out of the cells. Magnesium and manganese are essential to convert carbohydrates into energy for the brain.

**Cheat Sheet:** I put liquid minerals in my kid's juice, which is easy, and the minerals are undetectable. Get a good food-based vitamin, not one just cause it's your kids favorite cartoon character or because it has the most advertising. Go to your local health food store, ask questions, and read labels!

| VITAMIN | PURPOSE | SOURCE |
|---|---|---|
| A (Retinol) | Promotes healthy skin, bones, teeth, gums, eyes, urinary tract, and lining of the nervous, respiratory, and digestive systems. | Full-fat dairy products, fish liver oil, liver, eggs, butter, sweet potatoes, yellow and green vegetables. |
| B1 (Thiamine) | Required for carbohydrate metabolism and the release of energy from food. Helps your heart and nervous system function properly. | Whole grains and whole-grain breads and cereals, nuts, sunflower seeds, peas, potatoes, and most vegetables. |
| B2 (Riboflavin) | Promotes healthy hair, skin, nails, and tissue repair. Helps body cells use oxygen. | Liver, full-fat milk, cheese, eggs, liver, fish, poultry, almonds, and leafy green vegetables. |
| B3 (Niacin) | Helps maintain healthy skin and digestive tract and hormone production. Essential for cell metabolism and absorption of carbohydrates. | Lean meat, liver, whole grain and whole grain products, eggs, milk, nuts, potatoes, avocados, and soy flour. |
| B5 (Panthothenic acid) | Promotes healthy skin, hormone production, muscles, and nerves. Helps convert carbohydrates, fats, and proteins into energy. | Nuts, eggs, meat, whole-grain cereals, legumes, and green vegetables. |
| B6 (Pyridoxine) | For healthy teeth and gums, blood vessels, nervous and immune systems, and red blood cells. | Whole-grain cereals, liver, poultry, fish, meat, eggs, most vegetables, and sunflower seeds. |
| B12 | Helps prevent infection and anemia through the proper development of red blood cells. Aids the nervous system. | Fish, dairy products, meats, whole-grain breads, and eggs. |

| VITAMIN | PURPOSE | SOURCE |
|---------|---------|--------|
| BIOTIN | Assists the circulatory system and promotes healthy skin. | Eggs, liver, nuts, kidneys, and most fresh vegetables. |
| C (Ascorbic acid) | Vital for the immune system as well as for skin, bone, teeth, cartilage formation, and for wound healing. | Citrus fruits, tomatoes, raw cabbage, sweet potatoes, cauliflower, leafy green vegetables, peppers, broccoli, potatoes, strawberries, and cantaloupe. |
| D (Cholecalciferol) | Helps calcium to be utilized for bones and promotes a healthy heart and nervous system. | Fish liver oils, salmon, tuna, leafy green vegetables, mushrooms, eggs, full-fat milk, butter, and sunlight. |
| E (Tocopherol) | Promotes healthy cell membranes by helping to prevent the oxidation of polyunsaturated fatty acids in those membranes and other body structures. Aids fertility, stamina, and combating changes of old age. | Leafy green vegetables, wheat germ oil, olive oil, eggs, tomatoes, soy beans, brown rice, fresh nuts and seeds, and whole grains. |
| FOLIC ACID | Needed for the production of red blood cells and helps in the prevention of anemia, heart disease, and congenital abnormalities. | Leafy green vegetables, fruit, whole grains, liver, meat, poultry, fish, and full-fat milk. |
| K | Needed for normal blood clotting, healthy bones, and teeth. | Leafy green vegetables, cheese, liver, eggs, fish, full-fat milk, safflower oil, kelp, and raspberry leaf tea. |

| MINERAL | PURPOSE | SOURCE |
|---------|---------|--------|
| CALCIUM | For healthy bones, teeth, muscles, and essential for nerve message transmission. | Dairy products, soy (such as tofu), nuts, seeds, dried beans, leafy green vegetables, broccoli, and salmon. |
| CHROMIUM | Promotes the correct blood sugar levels and helps lower cholesterol levels. | Whole grains, brown rice, eggs, molasses, red meat, wine, bananas, lettuce, oranges, strawberries, apples, potatoes, parsnips. |
| COPPER | For the blood, bones, and nervous system. | Legumes, nuts, olives, and seafood. |
| IODINE | Regulates the thyroid gland. | All seafood, kelp, samphire, and iodized salt. |
| IRON | Essential in the formation of red blood cells and prevention of anemia. | Liver, red meat, eggs, dried fruit, asparagus, legumes, green vegetables, oatmeal, walnuts, sunflower seeds, and mushrooms. |
| MAGNESIUM | Essential for nerve and muscle function and maintaining blood pressure. | Dark leafy green vegetables, citrus fruit, nuts, whole grains, seeds, raisins, garlic, onions, potatoes, and chicken. |
| POTASSIUM | Needed for healthy bones, brain function, water balance, and fighting fatigue and muscle weakness. | Salmon, lamb, and all vegetables and fruits, particularly bananas, watermelon, and potatoes. |
| SELENIUM | Detoxifies arsenic and mercury and fights infections. | Whole grains, brown rice, Brazil nuts, seafood, eggs, and tomatoes. |
| SODIUM | Helps regulate the water in the body. | Salt and salty foods. |
| ZINC | Fights against infections and heavy metals, repairs wounds, and helps normal sexual functions. Needed for immune systems and enzyme production. | Seeds, nuts, whole grains, meat, eggs, brown rice, and berries. |

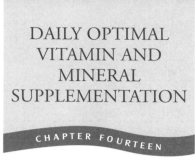

# DAILY OPTIMAL VITAMIN AND MINERAL SUPPLEMENTATION

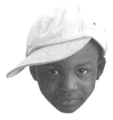

## CHAPTER FOURTEEN

**THE FOLLOWING RECOMMENDATIONS** for daily intake levels of vitamins and minerals are designed to provide an optimum intake range for maintaining good health. If possible, buy natural, organic vitamins, preferably labeled as not having sugar, preservatives, lactose, yeast, or starch. Also follow instructions regarding storage and recommended dosage. Some minerals and vitamins are toxic in high doses, and the safe dose can be exceeded if you take supplements from more than one source.

| VITAMINS | SUPPLEMENTARY DOSAGE RANGE |
|---|---|
| Vitamin A (retinal) | 5,000-10,000 IU |
| Vitamin A (from beta-carotene) | 10,000-75,000 IU |
| Vitamin D | 100-400 IU |
| Vitamin E (d-alpha tocopherol) | 400-1,200 IU |
| Vitamin K (phytonadione) | 60-900 mcg |
| Vitamin C (ascorbic acid) | 500-9,000 mg |
| Vitamin B1 (thiamine) | 10-90 mg |
| Vitamin B2 (riboflavin) | 10-90 mg |
| Niacin | 10-90 mg |
| Niacin amide | 10-30 mg |

| Vitamin B6 (pyridoxine) | 25-100 mg |
|---|---|
| Biotin | 100-300 mcg |
| Pantothenic acid | 25-100 mg |
| Folic acid | 400-1,000 mcg |
| Vitamin B12 | 400-1,000 mcg |
| Choline | 150-500 mg |
| Inositol | 150-500 mg |

| MINERALS | SUPPLEMENTARY DOSAGE RANGE |
|---|---|
| Boton | 1-2 mg |
| Calcium | 250-750 mg |
| Chromium | 200-400 mcg |
| Copper | 1-2 mg |
| Iodine | 50-150 mcg |
| Iron | 15-30 mg |
| Magnesium | 250-750 mg |
| Manganese (citrate) | 10-15 mg |
| Molybdenum (sodium molybdate) | 10-25 mcg |
| Potassium | 200-500 mg |
| Selenium (selenomethionine) | 100-200 mcg |
| Silica (sodium metasilicate) | 200-1,000 mcg |
| Vanadium (sulfate) | 50-100 mcg |
| Zinc (picolinate) | 15-30 mg |

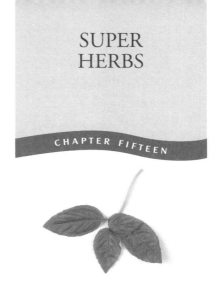

# SUPER HERBS

## CHAPTER FIFTEEN

FOR THOUSANDS OF YEARS, not just hundreds of years, herbs have provided a constant supply of healing agents to people. Whether from the roots, leaves, bark, flowers, or berries of plants, herbs have been scientifically proven to be nature's pharmaceutical agents as well as very effective in the prevention of illness. They are powerful, though usually gentle, and are a safe and natural alternative to drugs when used properly. You will find them packaged as teas, salves, tinctures, capsules, tablets, and concentrated extracts. Always follow the manufacturer's advice regarding the dosage.

**Cheat Sheet:** I believe herbs were given by God to bring healing to the body! My personal experience is that while they tend to move slower than medicine, the harmful side effects are not attached.

1. Aloe Vera. Internal and external; laxative, antiulcer, immune, antiviral, aids.
2. Bilberry. Diabetic retinopathy, macular degeneration, cataract, glaucoma, varicose veins.
3. Bromilene. Inflammation, sports injuries, respiratory tract infections, menstrual cramps.

4. Burdock. Mild detoxifier, promotes the production of urine and sweat.
5. Chamomile. Relaxing tea that aids digestion and the production of urine.
6. Dandelion Root. Liver disorders, water retention, obesity. Good source of potassium.
7. Dong Quai. Menopausal symptoms, premenstrual symptoms.
8. Echinacea. Viral infections, impaired immune functions, wound healing.
9. Ephedra. Asthma, hay fever, common cold, weight loss.
10. Fennel. Relieves cramps and gas.
11. Feverfew. Migraine headaches, arthritis, fever, inflammation.
12. Garlic. Infections, elevated cholesterol levels, high blood pressure, diabetes.
13. Ginger. Nausea and vomiting with pregnancy, motion sickness, arthritis.
14. Ginkgo Biloba. Decreased blood supply to brain, senility, ringing ears, dizziness, impotence, varicose veins, Alzheimer's disease.
15. Ginseng. Recovery from illness, stress, fatigue, diabetes, improvement of mental and physical performance, sexual function.
16. Golden Seal. Parasitic infections of gastronomical tract, infection of mucous membrane, inflammation of gallbladder.
17. Gotu Kola. Cellulite, wound healing, varicose veins, scleroderma.
18. Gugulipid. Elevated cholesterol and triglyceride levels, arteriosclerosis, hypothyroidism.
19. Hawthorn. Arteriosclerosis, high blood pressure, congestive heart failure, angina.
20. Hops. Cramps and gas.

21. Lapacho. Infections, *Candida Albicans.*
22. Licorice Root. Peptic ulcer, premenstrual tension syndrome, low adrenal function, viral infections.
23. Linseeds. Boost the liver with Omega-3 oils.
24. Lobelia. Smoking deterrent, expectorant in asthma, bronchitis, and pneumonia.
25. Milk Thistle or Silymarin. Liver disorders, hepatitis, cirrhosis of the liver, psoriasis.
26. Psyllium. Cholesterol.
27. Rosemary. Migraines, tension headaches, exhaustion, and fatigue.
28. Sage. Liver stimulant to promote the flow of bile.
29. Sarsaparilla. Psoriasis, Eczema, general tonic.
30. Saw Palmetto. Prostate enlargement.
31. Slippery Elm. Gentle laxative.
32. St. John's Wort. Depression, anxiety, sleep disturbance, aids in healing nerve damage, anti-viral.
33. Tea Tree Oil. Topical antiseptic, athlete's foot, boils, wound healing.
34. Turmeric. Inflammation, arthritis, liver, gallbladder.
35. Uva Ursi. Urinary track infections, water retention.
36. Valerian. Insomnia, anxiety, high blood pressure, intestinal spasm.

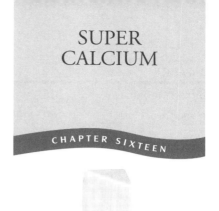

FROM THE TIME YOU WERE YOUNG, you were told that calcium is crucial for building and maintaining healthy bones and teeth. You may not have been told that it also plays an important role in the function of nerves, muscles, enzymes, and hormones. Calcium normalizes the contraction and relaxation of the heart muscles and protects against osteoporosis, rickets, and osteomalacia. Our need for calcium is critical during the growth years of infancy and childhood, but it is also important lifelong to keep our bones healthy.

Most plant foods contain calcium—spinach, watercress, parsley, dried figs, nuts, seeds, molasses, seaweed, dried beans, broccoli, and soy are all rich suppliers. Milk, eggs, salmon, and sardines are good calcium sources. Sea vegetables contain more calcium by dry weight than milk.

**Cheat Sheet:** You and your kids need calcium, and food is the best source. I like to add a dab of good cheese or a handful of sunflower seeds to all kinds of foods. It's easy! Be creative. Think healthy, not fat!

RDAs for calcium are as follows:

## INFANTS

| | |
|---|---|
| Birth–6 months | 360 mg. |
| 6 months–1 year | 540 mg. |

## CHILDREN

| | |
|---|---|
| 1–10 years | 800 mg. |
| 11–18 years | 1,000 mg. |

## ADULTS

| | |
|---|---|
| Men and women | 800 mg. |

## CALCIUM SOURCES

| Food | Portion | Calcium (mgs.) |
|---|---|---|
| Swiss cheese | 2 oz. | 530 |
| Jack cheese | 2 oz. | 420 |
| Cheddar cheese | 2 oz | 400 |
| Other cheeses | 2 oz. | 300–400 |
| Yogurt | 6 oz. | 300 |
| Broccoli, cooked | 2 stalks | 250 |
| Sardines (w/bones) | 2 oz. | 240 |
| Goat milk | 6 oz. | 240 |
| Cow's milk | 6 oz. | 225 |
| Collard greens, cooked | 6 oz. | 225 |
| Turnip greens, cooked | 6 oz. | 220 |
| Almonds | 3 oz. | 210 |
| Brazil nuts | 3 oz. | 160 |
| Soybeans, cooked | 6 oz. | 150 |
| Molasses, blackstrap | 1 tablespoon | 30 |
| Corn tortillas (4, w/lime) | 2 oz. | 125 |
| Carob flour | 2 oz. | 110 |
| Tofu | 3 oz. | 110 |
| Dried figs | 3 oz. | 100 |

| | | |
|---|---|---|
| Dried apricots | 3 oz. | 80 |
| Parsley | 1 1/2 oz. | 80 |
| Kelp | 1/4 oz. | 80 |
| Sunflower seeds | 2 oz. | 80 |
| Sesame seeds | 2 oz. | 75 |

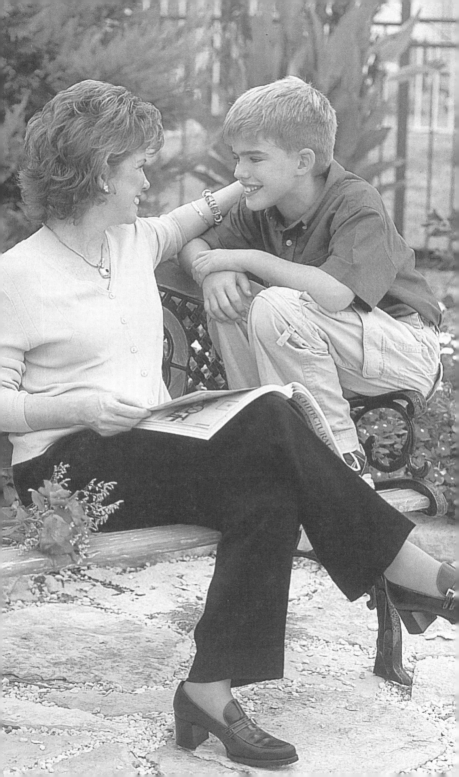

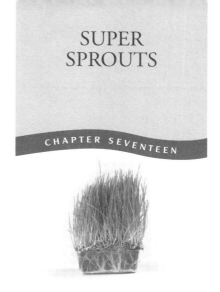

# SUPER SPROUTS

CHAPTER SEVENTEEN

THINK ABOUT SPROUTING SEEDS AT HOME. It's easy, it's fun, it's cheap, and it tastes good! Even the kids love them and love to grow them! They're great on sandwiches and salads, and they can be used as snacks as well. The rewards are great. They are loaded with trace minerals that are not so easily found in other foods. During germination all the nutrients needed by the young plant are mobilized from storage, which makes it highly nutritious.

You can get everything you need at your local health food store to sprout. You can purchase a commercial seed-sprouter, or do it cheaper with glass jars. To rinse the seeds, you'll need to cover the tops of the jars with cheesecloth that's attached with a rubber band. Find a warm, dark place for the seeds to germinate. You'll soak the seeds in water, then pour off the water through the cheesecloth and rinse the seeds. Keep the jar in a warm dark place, but rinse them two to three times daily until they are ready. The sprouts can be stored in a plastic bag or box for up to five days in the refrigerator.

**Cheat Sheet:** You can do it! Spouts are great to do with the kids, and they are an excellent way to get those needed trace minerals into the body.

| SEED | SOAK TIME (HOURS) | READY (DAYS) |
|---|---|---|
| Alfalfa | 6–8 | 5–6 |
| Chick Peas | 18 | 3–4 |
| Lentils | 10–15 | 3–5 |
| Mung Beans | 15 | 3–5 |
| Mustard | 6–8 | 4–5 |
| Radish | 6–8 | 4–5 |
| Sunflower | 10–15 | 1–2 |

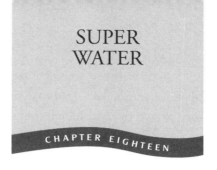

# SUPER WATER

CHAPTER EIGHTEEN

**WATER, WATER, WATER!** You can't get enough into your kids! Did you know that the body is 65 to 70 percent water? Even our bones are 10 percent water. And without water, there can be no life. This is because all the life processes—from taking in food to digestion to absorption to getting rid of wastes—require water. Water maintains homeostasis, or balance, in the cells, where everything is working correctly. Watery solutions help dissolve nutrients and carry them to all parts of your body. Through chemical reactions that can only take place in a watery solution, your system turns nutrients into energy or into materials it needs to grow to repair cells. Water is used for every enzyme process that governs the nerve chemicals, and therefore every thought and action, every chemical process, and therefore every function in the body.

Children need to drink more than adults, and the smaller they are, the more they need to drink. A boy between the ages of 11–14 needs to drink around 100 ounces of water per day, and a girl the same age needs eight 8-ounce glasses of water per day. As an adult, you should be drinking half of your body weight in ounces of water daily. For example, if you weigh 150 pounds, you should drink at least 75 ounces (a little more than one half a gallon) of water per day. If you are in hot weather or exercising or sweating for whatever reason, you need to increase these levels. Dehydration has been shown to contribute to poor concentration and memory.

I constantly stress the importance of drinking steam-distilled water. I know there is controversy over steam distilled, but I think it's the best water for your body. Some medical authorities think it throws off our biochemical/ electrical balance and prefer regular, purified water. Obviously, I don't agree. Because of its lack of minerals and flat molecular structure, distilled water draws other particles (nutrients and toxins) to it, which actually pulls out the toxins that build up in the body. Yes, you urinate more, but it's simply the bladder dumping more as the water pulls out unwanted substances. That's a good thing.

Here's another benefit of drinking distilled water. It helps rid the body of those awful cravings for junk foods. As the water flushes out your system, it cleanses the remainder of the junk food your kid may have eaten. Remember the last food eaten will be the next food craved. So if they've loaded up with junk, they will continue craving it if you do not get it flushed out of your system.

**Cheat Sheet:** Our family has been drinking distilled water for over twenty years. Our eight kids have had very few cavities and have been extremely healthy. We drink Clustered Water (see page 123) in the morning, for its wonderful properties, and on rare occasion drink bottled water when out and about. The little you invest in water will bring countless benefits to your body.

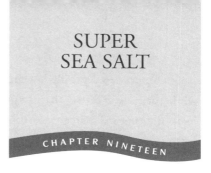

# SUPER
# SEA SALT

## CHAPTER NINETEEN

TABLE SALT, AS WE COMMONLY KNOW IT, truly deserves the horrible reputation it has gotten over the past twenty years and should not be used. Today, every common table salt sold is artificial. It is responsible for increasing blood pressure and heart problems.

But it is a mistake to confuse table salt with sea salt, which contains many health-promoting minerals such as magnesium, calcium, potassium, sodium, chloride, sulfate, phosphate, and many trace minerals. These trace minerals are absolutely vital in the electrolytic activity of the whole body, and without them you simply cannot function. Sodium helps convey energy and is the electrical charge that enables nerve impulses and muscle contraction.

Every day our body loses these vital minerals that must be replaced. And without salt you can't make adequate amounts of HCL (stomach acid), and in this weakened digestive state you can't absorb the minerals that are vital for activating enzymes and other important metabolic functions. Salt is also needed to maintain water balance within cells, control pH levels, and emulsify fats and fat-soluble vitamins. If you are avoiding salts, you may experience low blood pressure, dizziness, chronic fatigue, poor digestion, and hypo-adrenal function.

Americans typically consume 3 1/2 teaspoons of salt per day, while they could satisfy their requirements with 1/2 teaspoon. Keep in mind that 70 percent of this excess of table salt comes from processed foods.

Instead of avoiding salt, which is a healthy nutrient our bodies need, you need to go to a health food store and pick up sea salt.

**Cheat Sheet:** Make the switch—it's easy, inexpensive, and no one can taste the difference. But you will feel the difference, and you and your children's bodies will thank you.

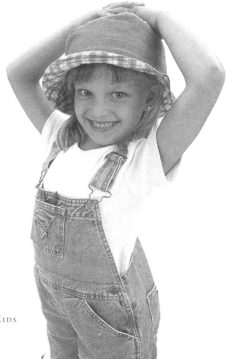

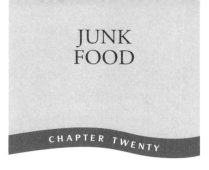

# JUNK FOOD

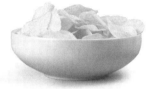

CHAPTER TWENTY

"JUNK FOOD" IS A GENERAL TERM that has come to encompass foods that offer little in terms of protein, minerals, or vitamins, and lots of calories from sugar or fat. We're talking about high-sugar, low-fiber, and high-fat foods that attract us and our children like magnets and put enormous stress on our healing system. While there is no definitive list of junk foods, most authorities include foods that are high in salt, sugar, or fat calories, and low nutrient content. The big hitters on most people's lists include fried fast food, salted snack foods, carbonated beverages, candies, gum, and most sweet desserts. The term "empty calories" reflects the lack of nutrients found in junk food.

According to a recent study in the *American Journal of Clinical Nutrition*, one-third of the average American's diet is made up of junk foods. Because junk foods take the place of healthier foods, these same Americans are depending on the other two-thirds of their diet to get 100 percent of the recommended dietary intake of vitamins and nutrients. Studies show that the average American gets 27 percent of their total daily energy from junk foods and an additional 4 percent from alcoholic beverages. About one-third of Americans consume an average of 45 percent of energy from these foods. Researchers are certain that such patterns of eating may have long-term, even life-threatening, health consequences.

If you have any question about the nutritional value of a food, judge it by the list of ingredients and the Nutrition Facts label found on packages. That label will list the number of calories per serving, grams of fat, sodium, cholesterol, fiber, and sugar content. If sugar, fat, or salt show up as one of the first three ingredients, you can probably consider that food to be a nutritional risk.

**Cheat Sheet:** Steer clear and don't give in to junk foods! "Do not crave [the king's] delicacies, for that food is deceptive" (Prov. 23:3). Food with no nutritional value can only cause harm.

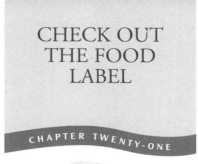

# CHECK OUT THE FOOD LABEL

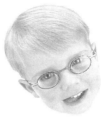

## CHAPTER TWENTY-ONE

MOST OF THE FOODS PURCHASED TODAY must carry a nutrition label. It's important that you understand what you're actually buying. Look at the "Nutrition Facts" on a product label for the specific information on such vital factors as nutrients, calories from fat, total fat, cholesterol, sodium, total carbohydrates, dietary fiber as well as the serving size. As you consider the calorie and fat values, make sure you understand the serving size. You may be surprised by what you find in what you were about to purchase.

Nutrient claims such as "low fat" can only be used if a food meets legal standards set by the U.S. government.

| | |
|---|---|
| Fat-free | Less than 0.5 grams of fat per serving |
| Low Fat | 3 fat grams or less per serving |
| Reduced Fat | At least 25 percent less fat per serving compared to similar food |
| Cholesterol-free | Less than 2 mg. cholesterol and 2 grams or less saturated fat per serving |
| Low Cholesterol | 20 mg. or less cholesterol and 2 grams or less saturated fat per serving |

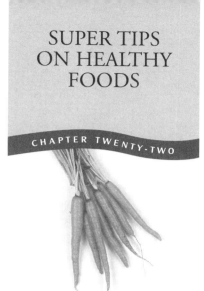

# SUPER TIPS ON HEALTHY FOODS

CHAPTER TWENTY-TWO

EAT AS MANY *fresh fruits and vegetables* a day as possible. By eating five per day, according to Johns Hopkins University, you can cut your risk of cancer by 30 percent and lower your systolic blood pressure by 5.5 points and the diastolic pressure by 3.0 points. Their researchers concluded that you could reduce your risk of heart disease by 15 percent and the risk of a stroke by 27 percent.

- Teas contain powerful antioxidants, are inexpensive, and easy to make. I get green tea and mix it with all kinds of other teas to make it tasty and fun. Get the kids involved. Tea is much better for you than some sugary soda or "so called" juice drink. At first you may need to add a little stevia or honey. That's okay. Keep blending until you find those that need no sweetener at all.

- Don't allow your child to leave the house in the morning without eating breakfast. And don't allow sugary cereals in your cupboards. There are all sorts of healthy, delicious, and quick alternatives.

- Researchers at Loma Linda University in California have shown scientifically that Kyolic® (a brand of garlic capsules found in any health food store) reduces the dangerous LDL levels of the blood and increases the beneficial HDL levels. A study in India showed that garlic has the ability to reduce blood clotting as well as serve as an anti-cancer agent.

■ Go to your local health food store and get a good powdered kelp to use for your seasoning. This is a great additive to your food as well as a plus to the thyroid, which controls your entire metabolism. A liquid bladder wrack—an old herbal remedy used for low thyroid—is also excellent when on a weight-loss program. It's very natural to the body and excellent for weight loss by speeding up the metabolism with no harmful side effects.

■ A good rule of thumb is to stay away from processed foods. Then you don't have to be concerned about those hidden ingredients labeled as "natural flavoring." Try to eat foods that are as close to the way that God created them—chemical free!

■ Go for foods rich in color! Stay away from the white deadly things! White sugar, white flour, white salt, even white potatoes. Choose red potatoes instead of white. Choose a dark lettuce or spinach instead of iceberg.

■ Eat small frequent meals, and make lunch you're biggest meal. Focus on foods that are high in protein and slow-releasing carbohydrates.

■ Go for Bible snacks instead of the processed foods. Fresh fruits, fresh veggies, nuts, raisins, granolas, yogurts, unrefined crackers, and flat breads—get creative! Genesis 43:11 specifically mentions pistachios and almonds. That's interesting in that those are particularly low in fat and calories. Nuts in general are a great snack food, with the exception of peanuts, which are really not a nut! Nuts are naturally rich in zinc, copper, iron, calcium, magnesium, and phosphorus, as well as being high in protein. Dr. Walter Troll of New York

Educate your children on what is good for them and bad for them. You may think they don't understand, but you'll discover they will learn faster than you. I knew it was working in our home when my seven-year-old Zachary said, "Don't eat potato chips, trans-fatty acids, bad for your brain." The Word says, "Train a child in the way he should go, and when he is old he will not turn from it" (Prov. 22:6). That training is for everything, including a nutritious diet.

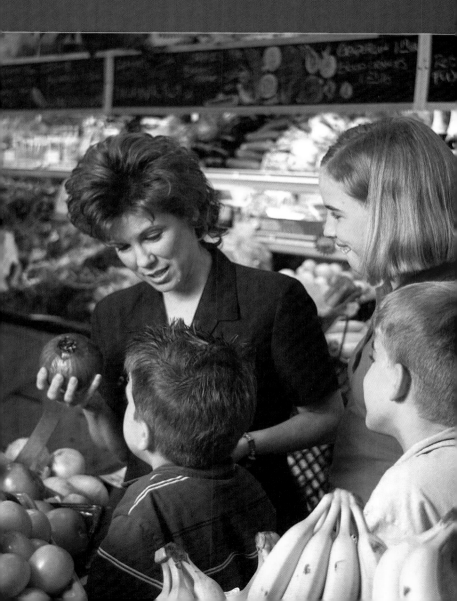

We use the 80/20 rule in our home. Eat the right food 80 percent of the time, and then you can splurge when it's a special occasion and not feel guilty. This takes away the condemnation and will help keep you from depriving yourself for long periods and then going on a binge.

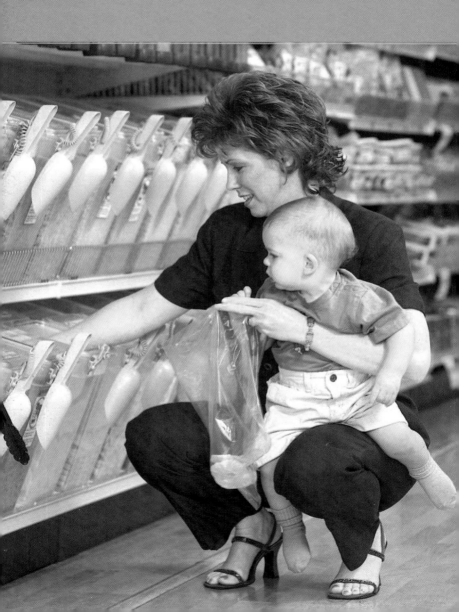

DR. VALERIE SAXION is one of America's most articulate champions of nutrition and spiritual healing and the mother of eight healthy children. A twenty-year veteran of health science with a primary focus in naturopathy, Valerie has a delightful communication style and charming demeanor that will open your heart, clear your mind, and uplift you to discover abundant natural health God's way. Her pearls of wisdom and life-saving advice are critical for success and survival in today's toxic world.

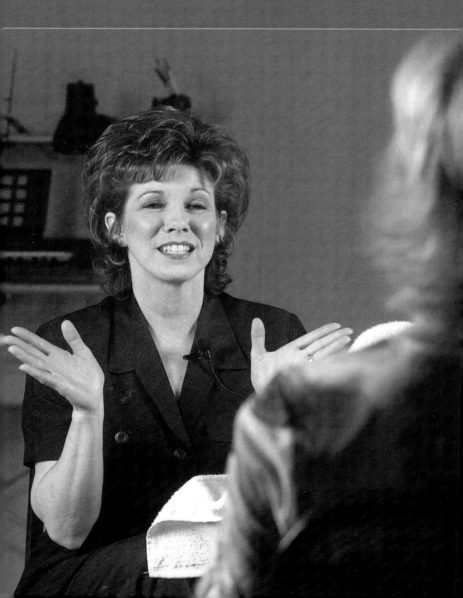

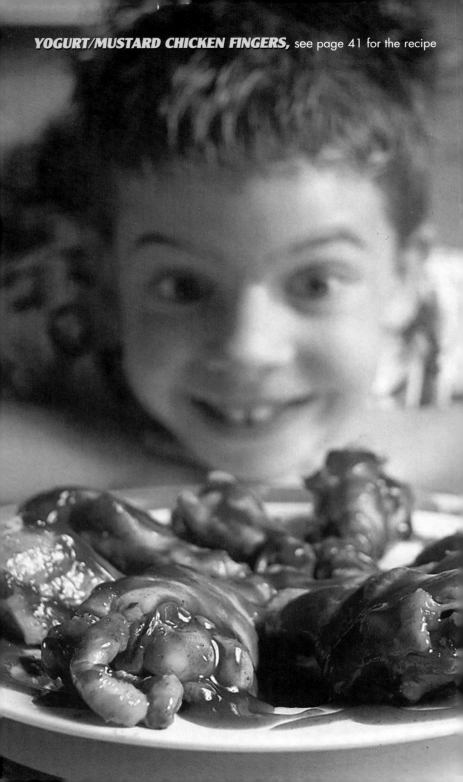

YOGURT/MUSTARD CHICKEN FINGERS, see page 41 for the recipe

University says that nuts are among the top cancer-fighting foods in the world, containing cancer blockers. Nuts also help to keep blood sugar levels steady so you don't get those bothersome hunger pangs that can lead you to grab the first snack you can find, which is normally high in sugar and carbohydrates.

■ Eat salmon instead of steaks or burgers. Try putting canned salmon bits on salads, bagels, or sandwiches.

■ If you must eat fast food, pass on the fried fish sandwiches. The fish is usually cod, pollack, or flounder—all low in good fat and usually fried in partially hydrogenated vegetable oil. It's better to go for the grilled chicken.

■ Sprinkle salads with olives, avocados, nuts, and sunflower seeds rather than bacon bits and croutons.

■ Dip your bread in extra virgin olive oil instead of marjoram or butter. Use butter as little as possible, and never use marjoram.

■ Read labels and be sure to never buy foods that contain partially hydrogenated or hydrogenated oils or with trans-fatty acids.

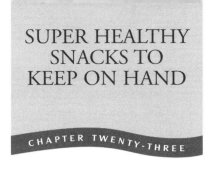

# SUPER HEALTHY SNACKS TO KEEP ON HAND

CHAPTER TWENTY-THREE

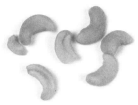

- Fresh fruit
- Seeds and nuts
- Carrot sticks and celery stalks
- Half an avocado with a squeeze of lemon
    and ground pepper
- Apples and small squares of cheese or cottage cheese
- Salads
- Boiled eggs
- Raisins
- Mashed bananas sprinkled with cinnamon
- Applesauce
- Live yogurt
- 100 percent rye crackers
- Chinese rice crackers
- 100 percent fruit chewy bars—I trust everything
    from Barbara's Bakery

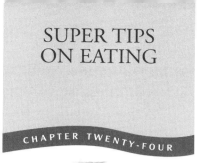

# SUPER TIPS ON EATING

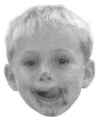

## CHAPTER TWENTY-FOUR

**BEFORE MEALS, EAT 4 OR 5 ALMONDS.** This will help to curb your appetite by sending a signal to the brain that you are full.

■ A good oat bran is a great way to end your day instead of a heavy meal at dinner. A half-cup a day has also been proven to cut your risk of cancer by 30 percent. It is very effective in the elimination of waste from the bowels, and we know that an unhealthy eliminative system makes for a breeding ground of disease.

■ Wait 10-15 minutes before having a second helping. This is how long it takes to get the signal to the brain to tell you you're full. In doing this, you usually won't want a second helping.

■ Sit down and relax while you eat. Purposefully slow down and don't overlap bites. You will be more aware of how much you eat and how full you really feel.

■ If you can avoid it, never eat past 6:00 p.m. in the evening! The later you eat, the less likely you are of burning it up. If you are having a smoothie, the time is not important because it is easily digested and absorbed.

- After your dinner, take the family for a brisk walk. Schedule in exercise three times a week. Remember there will never be a good time to exercise. You have to create one. At least 20 to 30 minutes is a good place to start. As with all changes in diet and exercise, consult with your physician first.

- If you have a problem with poor digestion, try a glass of steam-distilled water with a teaspoon of raw honey, a fourth of a fresh lemon, and two tablespoons of organic apple-cider vinegar. This mixture can be taken with each meal and has been proven to increase your digestive ability. Many of those with chronic upset stomach, acid indigestion, and gaseous problems find themselves being relieved with this inexpensive home remedy.

- Sampling food while cooking can be a real problem. Keep a dish of sliced fruit or veggies nearby to nibble on.

- A study was done of men from all around the world. Surprisingly, the healthiest men over all were French! Considering the typical heavy, sauce-covered French foods, this fact is quite shocking. The three things that made the difference in their diet were the following: a little red wine, which aids in digestion; lots of fresh foods and fresh herbs; and, most important of all, they ate their salad last. The living enzymes in the fresh vegetable eaten last works to break down all the other foods just eaten. It is an excellent palate cleanser, and because of that, it helps you to make the right choice in not choosing a dessert. With all your food being broken down more efficiently, you get better absorption of all your nutrients, you feel better, and you have more energy.

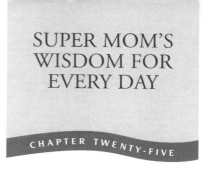

# SUPER MOM'S WISDOM FOR EVERY DAY

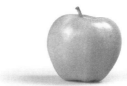

## CHAPTER TWENTY-FIVE

PEOPLE ALWAYS ASK ME how I handle my intense schedule while raising our eight children. The secret lies in making sure that everything regarding the children and schoolwork gets done in the evenings. That way you have help in the mornings, and the mornings are peaceful. I've tried it both ways and, trust me, this works.

I do three things in the evening!

- Lay the kids' clothes out the night before, and mine as well.
- Check homework and sign everything that needs to be signed.
- Prepare lunches.

You can also save yourself a multitude of headaches by going to the dollar store and stocking up on lunch containers. My kids bring them home . . . sometimes, so I get the cheap containers so it's not such a big deal.

Here's more wisdom for moms: Educate your children on what is good for them and bad for them. You may think they don't understand, but you'll discover they will learn faster than you. I knew it was working in our home when my seven-year-old Zachary said, "Don't eat potato chips, trans-fatty acids, bad for your brain." The Word says, "Train a child in the way he should go, and when he is old he will not turn from it" (Prov. 22:6). That training is for everything, including a nutritious diet.

Here's another point you may find helpful. We use the 80/20 rule in our home. Eat the right food 80 percent of the time, and then you can splurge when it's a special occasion and not feel guilty. This takes away the condemnation and will help keep you from depriving yourself for long periods and then going on a binge.

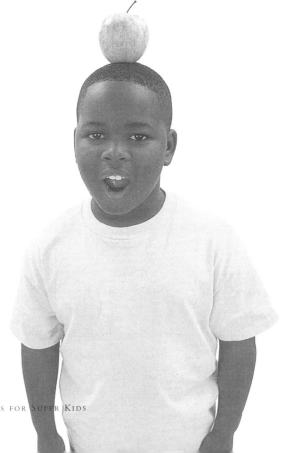

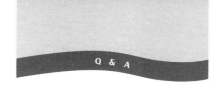

## Nutritional and Health Questions and Answers

DEAR DR. VALERIE, in your books and television appearances, you mention the importance of essential fatty acids for proper brain development in children. I'm confused. Aren't all fats to be avoided, especially since childhood obesity is epidemic in America today?

Good fats are a necessity. It is a primary focus of mine to make sure my kids get good fats on a regular basis. The brain is made of 60 percent fat, so the old saying, "You fat head," is actually a compliment. Without those good fats, the brain does not have the nutrients it needs to function. And as much as we need the good fats, that is how much we don't need the man-made bad ones. Please refer to Chapter 4 for the list of good fats and incorporate these into your diet.

DEAR DR. VALERIE, do you allow your children an occasional soft drink? Is it better to give them one that is artificially sweetened or one sweetened with real sugar?

Well, I do allow my kids to occasionally have a soda. We go for the real thing! While the sugar is not good and needs to be limited, the dangers of artificial, chemical-laden sweeteners are far worse than just having the real thing on a special occasion. I allow my children to have the clear sodas or orange soda. The reason is that while they are getting the sugar, they are not getting the caffeine. We also steer clear of food dyes. I can't go into all the side effects of artificial sweeteners, but I encourage you to check it out and stay away!

DEAR DR. VALERIE, my eight-year-old son has been diagnosed as hyperactive. The school wants him to be put on medication. Is there a safe and effective alternative that can make a difference?

Yes, and a million times, yes! You must change his diet and get to the root of why he is having these types of responses. In a study done on ADD and ADHD patients, *all* had an imbalance of essential fatty acids. When their level of good fats was increased, significant changes were made. Cleanse the bad; put in the good!

**DEAR DR. VALERIE**, my thirteen-year-old daughter started to menstruate this year and suffers terribly with PMS. Is there a safe and natural way to help her deal with this problem?

Immediately take her off any foods that are known to have added artificial hormones, such as milk, chicken, beef, etc. These absolutely throw off a young girl's hormones. Also stay away from foods served in plastic, which add zeno estrogen to the body. I have seen great improvement by cleansing the body, especially the liver, and supplementing daily with essential fatty acids. There is a reason they are called "essential."

**DEAR DR. VALERIE**, my daughter is suffering with acne. Is there anything I can do besides put her on birth control pills or Accutane? Our family doctor recommends these.

Once again, cleansing is essential! I see so many kids these days with bad complexions. They are in toxic overload. Yes, there are hormone changes going on, but even that will be greatly helped with cleansing and supplementing with herbal skin supplements and using natural products that don't strip the skin of natural oils. Essential fatty acids are excellent for not only the skin but also the brain and everything else you can think of. Lack of essential fatty acids is even linked to clumsiness!

**DEAR DR. VALERIE**, my sixteen-year-old son is a high school football player. He's recently begun a strenuous weightlifting program and has been taking a food supplement called Creatine. Is it safe for a teenager to take it? He says his coach is insisting.

While I love supplements and do sell them, I don't believe in pushing them, especially on kids. I have seen coaches push so-called healthy products for the single reason of getting a higher performance out of them for the sake of the team. I have major issues with that. Creatine is naturally occurring in the body, and many athletes supplement with it. However, my guess is that they have no knowledge as to how to take it. When combined with natural sugar, for instance, the body produces a substance called Creatinine, which can be dangerous to the kidneys or at least puts an extra strain on the kidneys. As with everything, get your facts straight and proceed with caution. Do it because it's good for you, not good for a game!

DEAR DR. VALERIE, at what age should I start giving my children vitamin and mineral supplements?

Immediately! The truth is that food is so depleted of nutrients that even if you are eating organic you are still not getting the vitamins and minerals you need. If you are eating non-organic, you are definitely in great need of supplemental help! Quick!

DEAR DR. VALERIE, is it possible for a child to have health problems that are directly related to Candida? Or is that something that doesn't happen until after puberty? The reason I ask is because my daughter has many of the symptoms you mention in your book, *How to Feel Great All the Time*, but she is only eight years old.

If they have been on an antibiotic, it is not only possible but highly likely! And if the mother had a yeast condition while pregnant, it is taken right into the child during the birthing process. It is never too early to begin adding good bacteria into you and your child. An easy way to do that is to eat yogurt daily, as much as possible, with live active cultures that are documented on the label. If any of my children are experiencing any area of compromised health, good bacteria (probiotic) are one of my first courses of action, and it usually nips any problem in the bud!

If you have searched in vain for answers to health problems such as PMS, headaches, chronic fatigue, skin rashes, or poor digestion, it may be due to an overgrowth of Candida or other yeast conditions. This parasitic yeastlike fungus will disguise itself in everything from athlete's foot to low blood sugar to obesity. It is estimated that over 90 percent of the U.S. population has some degree of Candida overgrowth in their bodies. I have written a booklet, *How to Stop Candida & Other Yeast Conditions in Their Tracks*, that covers the full scope of this problem.

**DEAR DR. VALERIE**, I read your book, *Every Body Has Parasites*. I know that you're absolutely correct about it. At what age should I begin a parasite cleanse with my children?

Don't cling to the notion that parasites are limited to the Third World. Parasitic experts estimate that there are between 100 and 130 common parasites being hosted in the American populace today, and a recent health report stated that 85 percent of Americans are infected with parasites. It is a lot easier to become a parasitic host than you think, and children are the easiest target! One would think that in a country where 50 to 55 million children are estimated to be hosts to some type of worms, regular screening for parasites would be a part of every medical checkup. But few health-care providers are taught to suspect, diagnose, or treat parasitic infections.

I recommend that a parasite cleanse usually start by the time children are two! They should definitely not eat meat before that, and when they do, it is time.

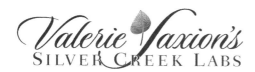

SILVER CREEK LABS

THROUGHOUT THIS BOOK, I have noted three specific products that will aid you in your efforts to provide your children with the essentials required to promote vibrant health. To order these products or to contact Silver Creek Laboratories for a complete catalog and order form of other nutritional supplements and health products, call (817) 236-8557, or fax (817) 236-5411, or write us at 7000 Lake Country Dr., Fort Worth, TX 76179.

Creation's Bounty. Simply the best, pleasant-tasting, green, whole, raw, organic food supplement available—a blend of whole, raw, organic herbs and grains, principally amaranth, brown rice, spirulina, and flaxseed. This combination of live foods with live enzymes assists your body in the digestion of foods void of enzymes. You will gain vital nutrients, protein, carbohydrates, and good fats to nourish your body and brain, resulting in extra energy and an immunity boost as well. It is a whole food, setting it apart from other green foods on the market.

Brain Sharpener is an herbal and natural combination shown to bring cognitive improvement, mental clarity, concentration, and creativity, enhancing optimum brainpower. Studies show that the ingredients in this proprietary blend may reverse age memory related problems, ADD, ADHD, Alzheimer's, Parkinson's, as well as other neurological concerns. The essential fatty acids in Brain Sharpener may reduce Cortisol levels, which is one of the main causes of depression, high blood pressure, constipation, stress, anxiety, insomnia, as well as vision impairment.

Dr. Lorenzen's **Clustered Water** is probably the greatest breakthrough in health science product development in this century. **Clustered Water**, produced at home using one ounce of solution to one gallon of steam-distilled water, replenishes the most vital support for all cellular DNA and the 4,000 plus enzymes that are involved in every metabolic process in your body. This amazing product increases nutrient absorption by up to 600 percent, which means your vitamins and organic foods will deliver far more vital nutrients to your body. It replicates the powerful healing waters of the earth! Excellent for cleaning out lymphatic fluids! It comes in a C-400 formula for those who are generally healthy and detoxed, and a SBX formula for the immune-compromised.

Three other products that you should strongly consider regard the cleansing of the body of Candida and parasites and toxins. Our **Candida Cleanse** is the most powerful natural agent I know of in the fight against Candida. A decade in coming, this is specifically formulated for total Candida cleansing. Candida may infect more than 80 percent of Americans, and the impact of a yeast overgrowth in young people can be significant. **ParaCease** is a powerful cleansing system the deals with parasites and Candida. It is made up of 25 unique, specialized ingredients that gently, safely, and easily cleanse the body and colon. **Creation's Cleanse** is an all natural, herbal cleanse formulated to address the body's seven channels of elimination: the liver, lungs, colon, kidneys, blood, skin, and lymphatic systems. It enhances the body's normal process of detoxification (ridding the organs of toxins) and cleansing (eliminating these toxins from the bowels).

*W*HEREVER SHE GOES, VALERIE SAXION constantly hears this complaint: "I can't remember when I last felt good. I'm exhausted and rundown. How can I start to feel good again?" This book is Saxion's response to that question, but it goes far beyond just feeling good. "So why don't you feel *great* all the time?" she asks. "Why are you willing to settle for less than 100 percent?" She then lays out a *Lifelong Plan for Unlimited Energy and Radiant Good Health* to help readers give their bodies the opportunity to start feeling great in four basic steps.

Specifically, Saxion guides her readers into an understanding of how their bodies work, how to stop eating junk food, and the importance of body oxygen, exercise, and water. *Candida*, detoxification, fasting, low thyroid, and weight loss are all covered as well as establishing a perfect diet that is filled with foods that supercharge the mind and body. Nature's prescriptions of vitamins, minerals, and herbs supplement all that she teaches.

Includes a state-by-state list of more than 800 of America's leading complementary alternative medical doctors.

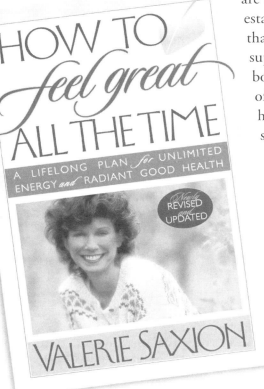

# NEW *from* VALERIE SAXION

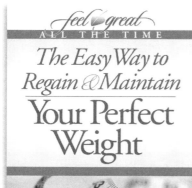

*feel great*
ALL THE TIME

*The Easy Way to Regain & Maintain*
## Your Perfect Weight

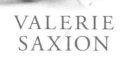

### VALERIE SAXION

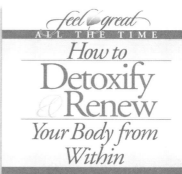

*feel great*
ALL THE TIME

*How to*
## Detoxify & Renew
*Your Body from Within*

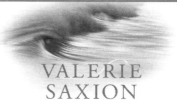

### VALERIE SAXION

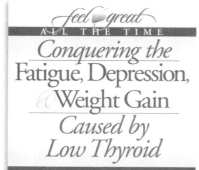

*feel great*
ALL THE TIME

*Conquering the*
Fatigue, Depression, *& Weight Gain*
*Caused by Low Thyroid*

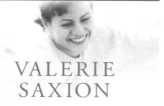

### VALERIE SAXION

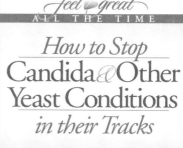

*feel great*
ALL THE TIME

*How to Stop*
Candida *& Other* Yeast Conditions
*in their Tracks*

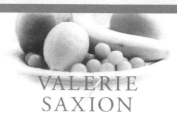

### VALERIE SAXION

Four powerful 64-page booklets in the *Feel Great All the Time* series.
If you need answers to these specific problems, and you need them
now, these booklets are for you! Valerie Saxion is one of America's
most articulate champions of nutrition and spiritual healing.

Do you have a chronic health problem that you just an shake off? Perhaps you have intestinal problems that come and go? ecurring bouts with diarrhea? Or you're tired all the time and feel epressed? Have you consulted with your doctor but not found an nswer? It is very possible that the cause of what you are experiencing directly due to parasites.

Don't cling to the notion that parasites are limited to the Third World. Parasitic experts estimate that there are between 100 and 30 common parasites being hosted in the American populace oday, and a recent health report stated that 85 percent of Americans re infected with parasites. The trick is that the symptoms caused by arasites are subtle because hey are experienced commonly by people without arasites, and the vast najority of health-care rofessionals have little raining in diagnosing hese masters of disuise and concealment.

If you're alive, you're t risk of this hidden risis that is damaging nillions of people eedlessly today. It s a lot easier to ecome a parasitic ost than you hink!

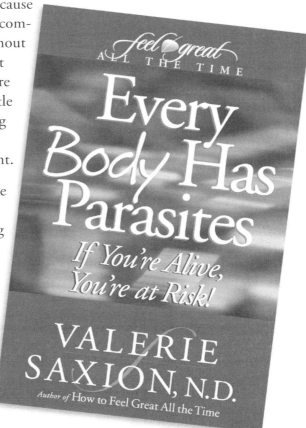

# Unleash Your Greatness

**AT BRONZE BOW PUBLISHING WE ARE COMMITTED to helping you achieve your _ultimate potential_ in functional athletic strength, fitness, natural muscular development, and all-around superb health and youthfulness.**

Our books, videos, newsletters, Web sites, and training seminars will bring you the very latest in scientifically validated information that has been carefully extracted and compiled from leading scientific, medical, health, nutritional, and fitness journals worldwide.

**Our goal is to empower you!** To arm you with the best possible knowledge in all facets of strength and personal development so that you can make the right choices that are appropriate for _you_.

Now, as always, **the difference between greatness and mediocrity** begins with a choice. It is said that knowledge is power. But that statement is a half truth. Knowledge is power only when it has been tested, proven, and applied to your life. At that point knowledge becomes wisdom, and in wisdom there truly is _power._ The power to help you choose wisely.

**So join us** as we bring you the finest in health-building information and natural strength-training strategies to help you reach your ultimate potential.

---

**FOR INFORMATION ON ALL OUR EXCITING NEW SPORTS AND FITNESS PRODUCTS, CONTACT**

**Strength & Honor**

BRONZE BOW PUBLISHING
2600 East 26th Street
Minneapolis, MN 55406

**WEB SITES**
www.bronzebowpublishing.com
www.masterlevelfitness.com

**612.724.8200**   Toll Free **866.724.8200**   FAX **612.724.8995**